REERS IN

THE HAIRDRESSING, BEAUTY AND FITNESS INDUSTRIES

CAREERS IN

THE HAIRDRESSING, BEAUTY AND FITNESS INDUSTRIES

eighth edition

Loulou Brown

KOGAN
PAGE

First published in 1980, author Alexa Stace, entitled *Careers in Hairdressing and Beauty Therapy*
Second edition 1983
Third edition 1985
Fourth edition 1988
Fifth edition 1990
Sixth edition 1993
Seventh edition 1996, revised and updated by Sheena Fitzsimmons
Eighth edition 2002, rewritten by Loulou Brown, entitled *Careers in the Hairdressing, Beauty and Fitness Industries*

Kogan Page Limited
120 Pentonville Road
London N1 9JN
UK

British Library Cataloguing in Publication Data

A CIP record for this book is available from the British Library.

ISBN 0 7494 3619 0

Typeset by Jean Cussons Typesetting, Diss, Norfolk
Printed and bound in Great Britain by Clays Ltd, St Ives plc

Contents

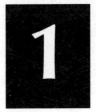

1

Introduction

Is this the job for you?

- ☐ Do you like working hard?
- ☐ Are you physically fit?
- ☐ Do you like people?
- ☐ Are you a sociable person?
- ☐ Do you like talking to people?
- ☐ Do you remain calm under stress?
- ☐ Do you like being with people?
- ☐ Are you self-motivated?
- ☐ Do you like hustle and bustle and being at the centre of things?
- ☐ Do you have a sense of humour?

If you've answered yes to all these questions, you should think about a career in the hairdressing, beauty or fitness industries. Although the hairdressing, beauty and fitness industries are three distinct professions, they are nevertheless closely linked. For example, if you are a hairdresser and work in a salon, as likely as not it will be a beauty salon and the people you work with will be beauticians, beauty therapists or make-up artists.

Masseurs are required in both the beauty and fitness industries, and the lead body for both the hairdressing and beauty industries is the Hairdressing and Beauty Industry Authority. All three service industries are geared to making their clients, both men and women, feel attractive and fit.

The three industries are expanding rapidly, particularly the fitness industry. This is because image and fitness are now perceived to be essential attributes for individuals, and also because there are so many exciting new trends in the industries. There is an increasing demand for good and well-qualified staff in all three professions.

As the required technology changes, so, too, do the qualifications demanded for the work. For example, the increasingly scientific approach to beauty has meant ever more electrical and electronic equipment to treat the face and body, and a beauty therapist must be thoroughly competent in handling this equipment. In hairdressing, an increasing number of people are having hair highlights or colours so the hairdresser must have a basic knowledge of chemistry to understand what happens.

All work in hairdressing, beauty and fitness involves providing a personal service. This means that your appearance and the way you behave towards your clients are crucial. It's not so much the qualifications, although they do help, but your appearance and behaviour towards others that will get you the work you are looking for.

Chapters two to six of the book outline the industries, the type of work available and set out details of how to find work and the relevant organizations. Subsequent chapters briefly outline the future of the industries and provide top tips on how to present yourself. There is detailed advice on how to apply for a job and an outline of the current legal provisions for both full-time and part-time workers, followed by details of training and training organizations. The Contact points chapter lists relevant organizations with details of how to contact them. This is followed by a brief reading list and an index.

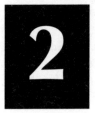

2 Hairdressing

Hairdressing is an expanding industry. In 1999 there were over 36,000 hairdressing salons (including some 5,400 that were offering beauty treatments). Nearly 90 per cent of the personnel who work in hairdressing are women, but the number of male hairdressers is increasing. Both men and women are now very aware of their image and the importance of their hairstyle. Hairdressing is, therefore, about much more than just a 'good cut'. Clients expect their hairstyle to project their individuality, make a statement about their lifestyle and contribute to a look that reflects their image.

Hairdressers should begin by talking at length with their clients. It is important to note the client's type and condition of hair as well as to take note of the particular views and specified requirements to project the required image. The accent is often on a natural look and a style that fits in with a busy lifestyle. As a hairdresser, you will be expected to give advice and help on how to create the desired image.

Hairdressers have to keep up with changing fashions in hairstyles, new ideas in colour concepts and developments in techniques and treatments. For instance, traditional barbering, involving 'scissors over comb' cutting and razor and clipper work, is an area in which there is increasing interest. In a large salon, there may be specialists who deal only with certain aspects of hairdressing. There may, for instance, be a hairdresser who only cuts hair, and someone else who only perms or colours hair. In a small salon, however, the qualified hairdresser will be expected to cope with whatever treatment the client requires. So, the smaller the salon, the more varied the work.

Hairdressers usually work a five-day week, but you may have to work six days a week, with either a fixed day off or working to a rota system.

Qualities required

Hairdressing is very much a personal service, so perhaps the most important requirement, apart from good hairdressing skills, is the ability to empathize with clients. Therefore, it is essential to have a warm, friendly and sympathetic manner. You may be brilliant with the scissors, but if you are curt and unfriendly towards your clients, they are unlikely to return. A hairdresser can quickly gauge whether or not he or she is successful by the number of clients who return regularly for their hairdressing appointments.

It helps if you have a calm, unflappable nature – tempers can run high in a busy, crowded salon – and the ability to talk easily to all kinds of people. You also have to be very patient, particularly when dealing with children who often object to having their hair cut and dislike sitting still for long periods.

You have to be good at working with your hands, and be both observant and interested in other people. Good health and stamina are important as the work is tiring and you will rarely be able to sit down. You will need to keep fit by taking regular exercise such as fast walking for 20 minutes a day or going to the gym at least twice a week, and by eating healthy foods. It helps, too, if you are of average height, as very tall and very short people will find the constant bending, stretching and reaching exhausting.

Personal appearance is very important. You should be well groomed and well turned out. The stylist whose own hair is a mess will not inspire confidence in a client. Hands should be clean and well kept, with no bitten nails.

No one with dermatitis is advised to consider a career in hairdressing as the somewhat stressful condition of work and the chemicals used are likely to aggravate the condition.

Types of work in hairdressing

General stylist/hairdresser

Trainees work towards NVQ/SVQ Level 2 in the salon. They are expected to work as part of a team assisting the senior members of staff. As a trainee you will be required to cut hair using basic techniques, perm and colour hair. Once you have achieved NVQ/SVQ Level 2, as a junior hairdresser you will have the opportunity of specializing as a colouring, perming or cutting technician.

Case Study

Shari Burnell is a stylist.

'I completed my NVQ earlier this year. The training was salon-based for four days a week and day release for one day to a training centre. The NVQ in hairdressing was at Levels 1 and 2; we also did beauty therapy at Level 1, which qualifies you to be a therapist's assistant. I did an adult training course over a year. I had started hairdressing as a school-leaver but never finished the course, so when my little boy was old enough to go to school, I decided to take it up again.

'The NVQ course was the quickest way for me to train and I could make use of my previous experience. I completed most of the theory side at home in my own time so that I could use the time at college on practical work. There are exams for the theory and your practical abilities are tested through continual assessment; for example, there were three assessments of blow drying a 'bob'. The training covers everything – cutting, colouring, perming and so on. We had training nights in the salon, which were very helpful. The practical side is the most difficult, especially the cutting, because it is so important to be accurate. You cannot afford to make mistakes: your clients are your income and you want them to keep coming back.

'Doing salon-based training worked out very well for me. It gave me lots of experience and Robert, the salon manager, took me on as a full-time stylist when I qualified. The creative and social aspects of hairdressing are what first attracted me to the career and what I enjoy most now. It can be difficult – you spend a long time on your feet and even if you are having an 'off' day, you still have to be cheerful with the clients. I'm beginning to build up my clientele now – it can take one or two years even in a town centre salon. One day I hope to manage my own salon.'

Technician

If you have had a good basic training and are already an experienced hairdresser, you might want to consider working as a technician, as the job commands a good salary. As a technician, your role will involve assessing, advising and carrying out a wide range of colouring, perming and remedial processes, and sometimes offering after-care guidance to clients. Outside of the salon, manufacturers employ technicians to work as trainers in their tuition centres or as field representatives, responsible for in-salon training and product/equipment testing. The minimum qualifications required are NVQ/SVQ Level 2, but Level 3 is preferred. You have to be well organized, full of confidence and be willing to travel a lot.

Lecturer/trainer

Many hairdressers combine part-time teaching with running a salon. Full-time teaching staff may spend around 20 hours per week teaching, with an additional nine hours on preparation, marking and assessment.

The minimum level of training required is NVQ/SVQ Level 3. It is also necessary to acquire a Further Education Teacher's Certificate to gain insight into how to teach and organize a class. A Post-Graduate Certificate in Education (PGCE) is preferred. You will be expected to attend continuing professional development courses to keep up to date with developments in the field. This ensures quality in the training that you give to hairdressers.

Freelance hairdresser

As a freelance hairdresser, you have to have a very thorough knowledge of hairdressing in all its aspects. You have to be self-motivated, well-organized, willing to undertake a very wide range of work, be willing to travel, as well as be able to work on your own without the need for talk and feedback from colleagues. You have to be able to deal with the unexpected, make decisions (and the right ones) quickly – and improvise where necessary.

The client potential is wide and varied. For instance, one day you may be working with an elderly disabled client in a hospital while the next you may be working with a model in a fashion show. Because you are freelance you will have to know a lot about business practices that relate to your work, such as book-keeping, stock control, accounting, etc, which may have to be carried out after 'normal' working hours. You may also need to acquire a comprehensive range of quality equipment and products for a 'portable' salon. The minimum qualification required is NVQ/SVQ Level 2 although Level 3 is preferred.

Salon owner

If you want to own your own salon, you have to be self-motivated. You also have to have extensive management skills and a lot of business knowledge, as well as be a very competent hairdresser. In addition to a day's work in hairdressing you have to undertake a lot of administration in the form of book-keeping, accounting, banking, stock control and conforming to the strict requirements of the health and safety regulations. You also have to recruit suitable staff and, most importantly, market your salon. The minimum qualification recommended to be a salon owner is NVQ/SVQ Level 3 but it is also advisable to have Level 4.

Case Study

Vicky is a hairdresser with her own salon.

'Being a hairdresser was all I ever wanted to do; I can remember being little and putting rollers in my grandmother's hair. I was always better at art than anything else at school.

'My first hairdressing job was when I was aged 13. I washed up, made coffee in a really trendy salon. I had a job in a salon straight after I left school. I trained for the City & Guilds NVQ Level 2 working in the salon. This meant two to three nights a week training with an exam at the end of it. I had to know about every basic haircut, health and safety, skin and ways of being polite. I was told how to dress. I was interviewed in the exam and had to know what to say and do. I was then sent to do courses with Wella and Sassoon and learnt to do colour work. I qualified at Level

2 when I was 19 and skipped ahead. I condensed the training into two-and-a-half rather than three-and-a-half years, and was then known as a young stylist.

'By the time I was aged 22 I was doing 45 clients a week, and I was exhausted. When I was about 24 I started to get restless. I didn't want 'team, team' any more. I went off to the States for a year and came back to work in the best salon in London. I wanted to do the thing I wanted to do, so I went out there and did it on my own. I wanted more variety.

'For 10 years I worked in about eight salons and was fully booked all the time. I retrained along the way, all the time – you have to – because of the new fashions and new techniques. Anyway, you are constantly learning – everything is about visual stimulation. You're in trouble if you only work in one place in one way.

'You have to be self-motivated. I didn't like being pushed into areas I didn't want to be in. I really love my work, which is cutting and colouring, but I have to do it in the sort of environment I want to be in. All I really wanted to do is to look after my clients. With them you have to have that slightly subservient, caring attitude. You've got to remain calm, laid back, even though things might go wrong.

'Now I have my own salon with a partner. My partner does the admin side; I'm useless at that. My Mum who's a book-keeper also helps. It's working out having my own salon. I work as hard as ever, even though I now don't have so many clients, but it's work I want to do.'

Specialist work

African Caribbean hairdressing

This is a rapidly expanding sector of the hairdressing industry with over 2,000 salons that cater for the technique. It requires specialist knowledge of the type of hair and extensive chemical knowledge. You also have to know about relaxing and pressing, as well as hair extensions, braiding, plaiting and African Caribbean finishing products designed for African Caribbean hair.

African Caribbean hairdressing is included in the NVQ standards. The minimum level required is Level 2, which includes perming, relaxing and neutralizing hair. Level 3 includes more specialized African Caribbean hairdressing skills and further styling techniques. There are a number of approved assessment centres across the country offering training in these techniques. For further information, contact The Caribbean and Afro Society of Hairdressers (see page 111).

Barber/men's hairdressing

Men's hairdressing in the UK has now become an art form, and there is great scope for creativity in this sector of the industry. Men's styles are now constantly changing and a wide range of skills are required. For example, the need for perming and colouring has dramatically increased. NVQ/SVQ Level 2 is preferred. Extra emphasis is placed on cutting 'scissors over comb', razor techniques and clipper work.

Specialist places of work

Armed forces

Stylists working in a military salon have to work flexible hours to suit their clientele. The minimum NVQ/SVQ level required is Level 2 but Level 3 is recommended as you will need to dress hair for the many formal occasions that are part of military life. Management skills are also required. Christmas and Easter are quiet times if you work in the armed services, and a base salon may close during these periods.

Cruise liners

Blow-drying and dressing hair are very important skills if you are going to work on a cruise liner. Hairdressing staff are expected to sell both hairdressing services and products to clients and will learn all aspects of business management and life aboard ship. Recruitment is strict and only fully qualified stylists are considered. The minimum training required is NVQ/SVQ Level 2 but Level 3 is preferred, and because hairdressing on cruise liners is very competitive, this is probably essential.

Steiner Transocean Ltd are the leading spa operator worldwide, and have spas on board over 100 cruise ships. They employ only fully qualified hairdressers and new employees are then trained up to Steiner's specific requirements.

Hospitals/care homes

These are often small units and have to facilitate disabled people. Health and safety regulations have to be strictly adhered to. Although most patients in hospital will require only a basic cut, blow-dry or set, long-term patients may want colours and perms. You have to be able to work in difficult surroundings, be especially sympathetic and understanding and have an awareness of the special needs of your clients. The minimum NVQ/SVQ requirement is Level 2 but it is recommended you also have Level 3.

Television and films

If you want to get a job in this elite part of the hairdressing industry, you have to have completed a full-time course in hairdressing, beauty therapy or make-up and be at least aged 21. The first six months' training is spent learning basic skills of TV make-up, period hairdressing, wig-making and other specialist skills. This is followed by six months on secondment to a make-up department before you become a full member working under supervision. Once trained, make-up designers are responsible for research, design and the execution of make-up and hair for all productions. You will need to work closely with lighting directors and set designers, as well as liaise with producers, directors, costume staff and artists. You will work long hours and must be willing to travel a lot. You must have a lot of creative imagination, a strong visual sense and a good degree of manual dexterity. Competition is intense for the limited number of jobs available so you have to have better qualifications than most people who apply. A minimum of five GCSEs is required as well as NVQ/SVQ Level 2, with a preferred two A levels and NVQ/SVQ Level 3. For further information, contact HABIA or Skillset (see pages 97–98 for training details).

HM prison service

There are only a limited number of hairdressing/training posts in the prison service, but training posts are expected to increase as more prisons introduce educational training programmes for their inmates. You will need a special strength of character, tact, ability to show sympathy for the inmates and awareness of their special needs. Hours of work are normally Mon–Fri 8 am– 4 pm. A sound basic training is required to become a prison hairdresser, including NVQ/SVQ Level 2, although Level 3 is preferred.

Getting work in hairdressing

Most hairdressers work in salons. Often salons carry notices of job vacancies in their windows, and you could just walk in one day and ask for a job. But do make sure to check out the salon first. Make sure you check the following:

◆ The salon must be easy to get to from where you live.
◆ If you are going to drive to work, make sure there are adequate parking facilities.
◆ Make sure the salon looks clean, tidy and well presented.
◆ Check the stickers on the windows that show the salon or staff are part of trade associations. A good salon should have a sticker with 'Nationally Approved Salon' written on it (see below). If the salon concerned is in any way connected to the following organizations listed below, this is also good news. It means that the owner has an interest in hairdressing beyond his/her own salon and that the salon has access to support and advice:

- NHF   National Hairdressers Federation;
- HEA   Hairdressing Employers Association;
- Guild   Guild of Hairdressers;
- CASH   Caribbean and Afro Society of Hairdressers;
- 365   a business club for salons, which involves owners and their staff in everything from business planning to personal motivation.

Nationally Approved Salons

A Nationally Approved Salon has met a number of standards. For instance:

- All the hairdressing staff working in the salon are qualified and/or experienced.
- All trainees are working towards qualifications.
- At least one hairdresser is State Registered (see below).
- All staff receive regular training to update their skills.
- The manager or owner has experience of running a business or is qualified to do so.
- The salon has public and treatment liability insurance.
- Current health and safety guidelines are followed in the salon.

If you choose a Nationally Approved Salon, you will work in a salon that appreciates your skills and expertise, and is prepared to invest in your future. Contact the NAS hotline number for details of an NAS salon near you: 01302 380029.

The Hairdressing Council

Those who successfully complete an approved form of training, for example, the NVQ Level 2 in Hairdressing, may apply to become a State Registered Hairdresser through the Hairdressing Council. Applicants must have at least six years' experience as a practising hairdresser, which may include periods under hairdressing training. Someone in an official position must certify the six years' experience. State registration costs very little and will provide you with the status of official recognition as well as other benefits. If you are registered with the Hairdressing Council this will provide proof that you are qualified and experienced in your craft.

Organizations connected with the hairdressing industry

- Hairdressing and Beauty Industry Authority (HABIA) – HABIA is recognized by the Department for Education and Employment as the national training organization for the hairdressing industry. The organization aims to improve upon and promote the already high professional standing of hairdressing through the development of high quality standards. It runs the NVQ/SVQ programmes jointly with City & Guilds and publishes a booklet entitled *Career Routes: The official guide to careers in hairdressing and beauty therapy.*

◆ Hairdressing Training Board (Scotland) – The lead body for hairdressing in Scotland.

◆ National Hairdressers Federation – Represents hairdressers and salon owners and self-employed hairdressers working in salons. There is a database of over 5,000 salons listed on the Web site.

◆ Hairdressing Council – A state-registered hairdresser is certified as competent to practise hairdressing. By the late autumn of 2001, the Hairdressing Council will have produced a handbook of hairdressers.

◆ Skillset – Skillset subsidizes a range of short courses for freelancers in hairdressing.

◆ Vocational Training Charitable Trust (VTCT)– This organization runs NVQs/SVQs in Hairdressing at Levels 1, 2 and 3.

3 Trichology

Trichology is the study and treatment of disorders of the hair and scalp. For instance, trichologists treat hair loss, which often responds to treatment, or there may be problems of the scalp, ranging from dandruff to more inflammatory conditions, which can be treated. There are often problems with hair texture, which may be caused by over exposure to heat or strong chemicals that can be treated by a trichologist.

Trichologists usually work in their own clinics, or in a clinic attached to a hairdressing salon, treating patients who come there direct or who are referred by their doctors or hairdressers. All hairdressers are expected to have some knowledge of trichology so that they can recognize disease or abnormal conditions and refer them for treatment, but trichology is actually regarded as a separate profession.

Local authority grants are not usually available for courses in trichology, though some students have successfully obtained discretionary grants, loans or sponsorship towards their study from various organizations. Some students have successfully applied for government-sponsored Career Development Loans. For further information about these loans, contact your bank manager.

Many qualified trichologists run their own private practices. Others are employed as consultants to industry and the legal profession, or in research and development for cosmetics and pharmaceutical companies. Some hairdressers take training in trichology as an additional qualification for their work.

Case Study

Renata Wink.

'Initially I trained in hairdressing through an apprenticeship with day release to college. It was the theory and science classes at college that really stimulated my interest in the hair and scalp. I practised as a hairdresser for a number of years, taking the City & Guilds Advanced Hairdressing qualification (Level 3), followed by a teaching certificate. There wasn't a great deal on the subject of trichology in any of these courses, but there was enough to feed my interest and spur me on to find out about training and qualifying in trichology.

'The Institute's course is normally for three years but I was exempt from the first year because of my hairdressing teaching certificate. It really is a lot of hard work and you need to be very committed and self-motivated to succeed – it occupied virtually all my free time for two years.

'Clinical experience is an essential element in the training. I was lucky enough to be employed at the Scalp and Hair Hospital in a full-time post for 16 months. I feel that I benefited enormously from doing more than the minimum observation. Personally, I don't think you can ever do too many hours. There are so many hair conditions – so much to see and learn; one condition can look totally different on two different people.

'I started up my own clinic, based at a private health centre, and, so far, it's doing quite well. Some people come to me after being referred by GPs or hairdressers or through the Institute when people ring to find out their local practitioner; others refer themselves because they know I'm there.

'I find the whole subject fascinating and I think that technical interest in the subject is important. Anyone wanting to do trichology should also be able to assess and analyse information from clients. For example, someone might be convinced that a hairdresser has damaged their hair, but the actual causes might be totally unrelated.

'You've really got to like working with people and want to help them. Being able to treat and advise a patient is immensely satisfying, but many of the hair and scalp conditions are very distressing for people so good counselling skills are important in this job.'

Contact the Institute of Trichologists for further information. (See pages 98–100 for training details.)

4 Beauty

Most people think that working in the beauty industry means working in a salon, dabbling with cosmetics. In fact the work covers a much wider field and is very much more demanding. The work is challenging and you need stamina as well as a good level of education. The training is much more rigorous than you might suppose; it cannot be considered a soft option.

Thorough training and many qualifications are essential for practising professionals over a wide range of subjects. For instance, study is included on science, diet, exercise and nutrition and you have to keep abreast of the ever-increasing technology introduced into the industry. This is a caring profession, requiring individuals who are patient with, and caring of, other people.

There are many job and career possibilities if you are interested in the beauty industry. If you want sound training in the full range of beauty treatments, which includes make-up, facial and body massage, electrical epilation (removal of unwanted body hair) and slimming treatments, you would do best to take a beauty therapy course. If, however, you are fairly self-confident and interested in selling, you might consider work as a beauty consultant in a department store. There are also other specialisms such as manicure and make-up, but on their own these offer limited employment opportunities, so it is advisable to take one of these specialist courses as an additional qualification or as part of a broader course.

Although most courses are open to both sexes, jobs may be

open only to women as beauty salons can claim exemption from the Sex Discrimination Act. Almost all those involved in careers in the beauty industry are women. All the main areas of the beauty industry are outlined below together with a number of specialist areas.

Types of work in the beauty industry

Aromatherapy

Aromatherapy is used both to alleviate many symptoms of illness and promote well-being and good health. It is the therapeutic use of essential oils, the aromatic essences of which are believed to contain medicinal properties and natural healing powers that improve the balance of mind and body. The essences are extracted from large quantities of parts of medicinal and aromatic plants, flowers and trees. Once absorbed through the skin they work rapidly. They are diluted in vegetable oils such as almond, sunflower, wheatgerm, avocado or alcohol, and may have calming, toning, regulating or stimulating effects.

Essential oils are powerful chemicals and if used to excess may prove dangerously toxic. It is therefore essential to have proper training. The Aromatherapy Organizations Council (AOC) has a number of member associations with accredited schools. Contact the AOC for further details. See also the CIDESCO Diploma on page 69.

Beauty therapy

The work covers a wide spectrum of activities. Beauty therapists are trained to be able to offer a wide range of treatments for the face and body. Some of these treatments are designed to improve the texture and appearance of the skin; others are concerned with body shaping and fat reduction.

You need to be able to analyse a client's skin condition and offer appropriate treatments. For example, some people may need treatment for acne while older people and clients with drier skins may need treatments that hydrate and nourish the skin. Facial treatments include make-up, cleansing, toning, applying face masks and facial massage; electrical treatments, for example, steaming to alleviate greasy skin; use of electronic instruments to tighten the muscles in the face; and eye care, including lash and brow treatments. More specialized treatments might include cosmetic camouflage, which involves blending make-up to match skin colour to cover scars, birthmarks or blemishes.

All therapists must be able to perform facials, body massage, wax treatments, eyelash tinting, manicures and pedicures (hand and foot care). The title aesthetician or aestheticienne is sometimes used for a beauty therapist who is trained in body massage. Many beauty establishments offer the related services of aromatherapy and body massage. Training in all these specialized skills is essential.

Beauty therapists may also offer depilation (temporary removal of hair using wax and other methods), heat treatment and figure correction/slimming treatments. There are special qualifications in electrical epilation, which is the permanent removal of superfluous hair from the face and body.

Beauty therapists work in beauty salons or clinics in health and fitness centres, or on health farms, passenger liners, department stores, etc. They may also be self-employed, either in their own salons or making home visits to clients. In 1999 there were over 4,800 beauty therapy salons and over 800 beauty therapy salons within other businesses, for example hotels or leisure centres. Over 99 per cent of all staff working in beauty therapy are female.

Some beauty therapists work in hospitals performing electrical epilation as dermatologists' assistants, carrying out cosmetic camouflage together with plastic surgeons or giving facial treatments specifically to help the recovery of mental patients. Beauty treatments are sometimes used to help in the treatment of psychiatric patients, and some therapists can find employment in hospitals and clinics working with dermatology or plastic surgery patients using cosmetic camouflage techniques to help build morale.

A beauty therapist needs to be very patient and understanding of his or her clients' needs and should be well groomed. You may have to deal with people who are embarrassed, nervous or suffering from stress. It is important to have a confident manner when handling complicated machinery or instruments so that you can help to overcome clients' fears and persuade them to relax.

If you are working with cosmetics, it is important to have a good sense of colour. This is particularly important if you are involved with cosmetic camouflage work.

The wide range of treatments demands an extensive knowledge of anatomy, physiology, nutrition and cosmetic science. Sometimes a client may be suffering from a condition that requires medical attention. As a beauty therapist, you will have to be able to recognize such a condition and refer your client to a doctor. You will also have to decide when a course of treatment should be carried out, with the prior approval of the client's doctor.

Wherever you wish to work, and whatever area you wish to specialize in, if you want a sound training in the full range of beauty treatments, it would be best to take a beauty therapy course. An NVQ/SVQ Level 2 in beauty therapy is the accepted starting qualification of a beauty therapist, but salons would expect their staff to attain NVQ/SVQ Level 3 and do not normally employ beauty therapists without this qualification. You will be expected to work as part of a team and will be required to assist therapists with treatments and support health and safety in the salon. If you have NVQ/SVQ Level 3 in beauty therapy, you should have the ability to carry out the full range of treatments.

Other relevant qualifications listed in this book are the CIDESCO International Diploma Course (pages 70–71), the CIBTAC Beauty Therapy and Electrolysis Course (page 72) and the ITEC Aestheticienne Diploma, the Diploma in Physiatrics, and the Beauty Therapy Diploma (page 73). There is also the Edexcel BTEC National Diploma in Beauty Therapy (see page 74).

Case Study

Bev Stocks *is a beauty therapist in a high street hairdressing salon.*

'I've been here 12 months now. It is wonderful to work alone and have responsibility for the beauty salon. Although it is owned by the hairdresser, I am my own boss to a large extent. I do facials and massage, manicure, pedicure, waxing, eyelash and eyebrow tinting and shaping, and also electrolysis, which required a separate certificate. As a beauty therapist I think you really need to be able to do electrolysis as a "bread and butter" line. It can take 12 to 18 months to treat an area so your customers return for treatments, giving you a regular client base. The electrolysis I do is for the permanent removal of hair but it is also used for treating red veins, etc, for which you need an advanced certificate. I intend to take the extra qualification when I have time to do the training.

'The things I enjoy most about this job are meeting people and seeing the results of my work. For me it is most rewarding to treat people with problems. Clients come in with badly bitten nails, unwanted hair or whatever, and if I can provide a treatment and send out a happy client an hour later it makes me feel really good.

'I first chose beauty because I wanted a job that involved helping people. I talked myself out of nursing when I had thought about the pros and cons. Beauty seemed a bit more glamorous, but it isn't as glamorous as most people think. It is hard work. Many people think you "just do make-up", but the training is very demanding involving in-depth study of anatomy and other relevant sciences. You don't need all that to "just do make-up". I took a three-year combined hairdressing and beauty course at the local technical college, which led to City & Guilds qualifications in hairdressing, beauty therapy and electrical epilation. I always preferred beauty to hairdressing. I think you have more autonomy – a client comes in for their legs waxing and it is up to you to decide how to do it; in hairdressing you are directed by the customers to a greater extent.

'It is a bit of a 'Catch 22' when you first qualify as you cannot find a job because you don't have any experience and cannot gain the experience until you have a job. At first I worked as a beauty consultant, which gave me sales experience – there is some selling of products in most therapy jobs – and experience of advising clients. This was enough to get me into a salon. I worked in a hair and beauty salon for six years before coming here. The business here is still developing, so it is very exciting. I consider myself lucky to be one of the few people who actually looks forward to coming to work every day.'

Body treatments

Some beauty therapists are qualified in aromatherapy (see above) and are able to treat people who suffer from stress and tension. A high level of training is required together with a good knowledge of all the essential oils, their properties and their effects on the body. Body massage is normally carried out manually, although there are some treatments that use machines. As a beauty therapist, you will need to have a thorough under-standing of anatomy and physiology and of the effect of massage on clients with high blood pressure and back problems. Some massage treatments are concerned with lymph drainage, which helps to remove wastes and toxins from the body. For further details about massage, see Chapter 6, page 46.

Many salons offer a range of body treatments using various types of machinery. There are, for example, pads that are applied to areas of muscle to give physical contractions, known as faradic treatments. There are also treatments for cellulite (a condition that makes the skin look dimpled like orange peel). These include galvanic machines and other electrical slimming machines that provide a vigorous massage. Also, machines with a vacuum suction device help to break down fat to aid lymphatic drainage. Other body treatments may involve using products containing seaweed or mud that help the body to slim.

It is a good idea to have at least the NVQ/SVQ in Beauty Therapy at Level 2. Other training includes CIBTAC's Body Therapist Diploma course and the VTCT's Foundation Course in Anatomy and Physiology and the Diploma in Anatomy and Physiology (see pages 74–75).

Beauticians

Beauticians specialize in skin care. The work includes cleansing the skin, make-up, removing blemishes and helping the client to counteract the effects of tension and fatigue. This includes massage of the face, either by hand or electricity, removal of superfluous hair, manicures and pedicures, shaping eyebrows and colouring eyelashes, acne and open pore treatment, make-up for special occasions and make-up lessons. In a large establishment there may be beauticians who specialize in electrolysis and manicure.

The work of the beautician and of the beauty therapist often overlaps, but beauticians are not concerned with body treatments (see above), and their training does not include such an exacting knowledge of anatomy and physiology.

The beautician works in a salon, which may be part of a larger establishment – beauty salons are now to be found in hairdressing establishments, department stores or in the growing number of health farms and health clubs.

You will need to have a calm and even temperament, a cheerful, outgoing personality and a well-groomed appearance. You don't have to be young and beautiful (many employers prefer their staff to be mature and older) but you do need to pay attention to your appearance. You have to be fit and well groomed, and in this business it helps to have supple, well-kept hands. Your manner should be positive and reassuring to inspire confidence in your clients.

CIBTAC offers a Beautician Diploma and ITEC offers specialist courses for beauticians (see pages 76–77).

Hair removal

Depilation (temporary hair removal) involves using wax or sugaring to remove hair from legs, arms, the bikini line, underarm and face. Sugaring is a comparatively new technique using sugar to remove body hair from the follicle. A paste made from sugar, water and other ingredients is applied and then removed together with the superfluous hair. Practitioners may be self-employed or work in a salon where they may also use other depilation and epilation (permanent hair removal) methods.

NVQ/SVQ at Level 2 in Beauty Therapy is preferred. IHBC and CIBTAC have qualifications with units for sugaring.

Make-up artist

Make-up artists carry out a whole range of tasks from tidying hair and powdering television presenters' faces in order to stop shine, to creating realistic-looking scars and wounds, creating make-up and hair for historical characters, and ageing characters through the course of a film or series. Artists need skills in using many different materials, such as latex and plastic, as well as make-up. They also deal with performers' hair and look after and maintain, repair and dress, wigs and hairpieces, so hairdressing is a major part of the work.

All make-up artists have to be able to administer make-up to clients, often called a makeover. This may include make-up for photographic sessions, corrective make-up for blemishes, or make-up for special occasions. There are opportunities for make-up artists in beauty salons and in hospitals, with clients following injury or surgery, and with people wishing to work in the television and film industries. You must have a strong visual sense and a creative imagination and be proficient in all aspects of make-up. You will need to work meticulously and patiently and be able to work as part of a team, communicating with many different sorts of people. For example, you will need to work closely with hairdressers, photographers, fashion designers, lighting directors and set designers. The hours are long and you will need to be very fit and have an enormous amount of stamina as you can expect to spend a lot of time on your feet. Your day will begin early, maybe as early as 4 or 5 am. You should also be willing to travel and live away from home. Most of the opportunities for make-up artists are for freelancers.

This is a very competitive field so it is a good idea to be well trained. An NVQ/SVQ Level 3 in Beauty Therapy is recommended. If you apply to TV companies, they may want you to have A levels. There may be opportunities for training in make-up for film and television through the Skillset National Training Organization scheme run with the British Film Institute (see page 78). The London College of Fashion runs a specialist course in Theatre Studies (Theatre Make-up Option). See also the CIDESCO Diploma in Make-up (page 77).

Case Study

Wendy *is a freelance make-up artist. She has worked all over the world with many photographers and clients in the music, film, television, advertising and fashion industries.*

'I've always been interested in fashion, music and film. I wasn't sure what that entailed, but at school I studied art. I did a course at the London College of Printing that involved work placement. I didn't enjoy this much at the time but in retrospect, I realised how much I learnt and how valuable it was. I learnt about basic photography and this enabled me to develop ideas and pictures of my own. I started a job as a paste-up artist and slowly moved on to print production. But I quickly became frustrated with the lack of creativity. I became disappointed with everything and decided to travel. To make money I temped.

'I had a friend who was a session hairdresser in Paris. He suggested I try working as a make-up artist. I found a private college course where I learnt the basics of make-up for two months: hairdressing, fashion, film, prosthetics and black and white make-up. I had to complete both written and practical exams. In addition, I had to work on photographs for a portfolio, and this resulted in a diploma. Then I travelled to Paris and assisted my hairdresser friend for three months, all of which I hated. I had no money and was very lonely. After coming back to London, however, I realized how much I had benefited from my miserable Paris experience.

'My first job in London was with a school friend's band doing their pop video. I did not realize how long the hours would be and how hard the work was. All along, I had to be supported by benefits to survive. Nevertheless, I decided that make-up was for me and that I was going to take it seriously. My next step was to visit model agencies to test, that is, to take photographs of models I'd made up to put in my book, my portfolio. I went to make-up agencies and was told to write a letter to everyone I wanted to assist and work with. As an assistant you clean the make-up artist's brushes and learn from watching. It is really down to you at the end of the day – you can't learn this work at college.

'My next step was to get an agency to find work as a fully-fledged make-up artist. It's quite hard to get an agency but eventually I did; it was the only way to get into magazines. I was still assisting well-known make-up artists at the same time.

'You have to get known and perform well under pressure and have very good social skills – and you have to be very fit; at one point I was working out daily. To get on you have to take risks, always be looking at all the areas of work you want to be in, and be hungry for the work. At one point I was doing three shows a day, making up four to five models per show. The more you do the faster you become. Your techniques become better. It's the same make-up adapted for each girl. It's quite a mothering role because models feel very vulnerable without anything on their face – and they are often very lonely; you have to be very understanding.

'After a while I started to make a bit of money. You always have to be careful about the cash flow – often there isn't any. You can't walk off the job and you can never be sick. All the time you have to think 'I will not let this beat me'. I really don't think people took me seriously when I started; I made them take me seriously. There is stubbornness in me and I'm determined to get to where I want to be.

'I travel back and forth to Paris. I have an agent in London, one in Paris and one in New York. I don't get much notice to do a job. Each job looms for about a week. I will decide with my agent about whether it's good for me or whether I want to do it, before I confirm the option. I'll probably be sent a fax the day before, or a couple of days before if it's abroad, telling me the call time, the location, how many models and who is working on the job. I'll arrive with my kit, look at the clothes, and speak to the stylist to see what he or she expects and the photographer to find out what style of photos he or she is going to take. Then I'll get on with it. If you're travelling abroad, it's weird. You pick up your tickets and go! I once went to Zanzibar. I had three days' notice.

'I think what is important is hands-on experience and whom you know, not qualifications. The work you do has to come from inside. It's not a head thing; it's a feeling.'

Manicure and pedicure

Manicures involve filing and shaping the nails, removing cuticles, applying creams and applying nail polish. Pedicures are similar to manicures but are for the feet. Foot massage may be applied as well as the removal of hard skin.

It is a good idea to aim for at least the NVQ/SVQ Level 2 in Beauty Therapy and there are a number of courses that specialize in both manicure and pedicure. For instance, City & Guilds run an NVQ in Manicure. The International Health and Beauty Council, CIBTAC and ITEC offer separate Manicure Certificates.

Nail extensions

Nail extensions are artificial structures applied to the natural nail bed to enhance the appearance and length of the natural nail. Salons now often offer 'nail art', which involves a great deal of artistic flair and skill. Air brushing is a very popular treatment and nail jewellery is very much in demand, that is, having diamante and pendants fixed on to the nails. To become a nail technician, artistic flair and skill are essential as well as thorough training. You will need to be well organized, self-motivated, willing to travel and have a good creative imagination. There are opportunities available in hairdressing and beauty salons and there are an increasing number of nail technicians working free-lance.

The preferred qualification required is an NVQ/SVQ Level 2. CIBTAC offers Nail Treatments and Nail Technicians courses. Further information from the International Nail Association or CIBTAC.

Electrolysis

Electrolysis is the removal of superfluous hair from the face and body using electricity. It is the only method of permanent hair removal. A fine needle is inserted down the hair follicle to the base, which is cauterized by a mild electrical current. Specialized training is essential for all electrolysis work, which is usually done in clinics.

For details of training, contact the Institute of Electrolysis (see pages 79 and 105). There is an NVQ Level 3 in Electrical Epilation and CIBTAC provides a Beauty Therapy and Electro-lysis course as well as a Diploma in Electrolysis (see pages 72 and 80). There is also the CIDESCO Diploma in Electrical Epilation (see pages 79–80). Edexcel provides courses within BTEC National and Higher National Certificate schemes.

Hydrotherapy

Hydrotherapy is using water, either externally or internally, to cleanse and revitalize the body and maintain or restore health. Many salons and health spas offer hydrotherapy treatments. These may be, for example, in the form of high-powered jets with strong streams or sprays of water that stimulate the circula-tion and ease muscular pain. Jacuzzis are used in hospitals to relieve pressure sores and for bedridden patients. Colonic irriga-tion, consisting of water at body temperature being injected into the rectum, clears the colon of poisons, gas, accumulated faecal matter and mucous deposits. Thalassotherapy uses seawater or seaweed that induces sweating, thus cleansing and toning the skin and lymphatic system. For further information, contact HABIA or the Association and Register of Colon Hydrotherapists (see page 106).

Beauty consultant

The main work of the beauty consultant is to sell the products of cosmetics houses. Consultants work mainly in department stores where they stand behind the counter giving advice on make-up and skin care to customers. You have to be completely familiar with the firm's range of products and must have the confidence and self-assurance to deal with any customer, however difficult.

Demonstrating products may involve doing makeovers for customers. Consultants encourage customers to buy the products that have been used. The work also includes general retail duties, such as dusting displays, organizing stock, arranging displays and 'testers', as well as handling payments.

The consultant usually works on a basic salary, plus commission, and future promotion depends on sales. If you prove to be good at sales you may eventually be promoted to senior consultant, with the job of visiting the various stores to supervise the other consultants, training newcomers and making sure that their counter displays and personal appearance are up to standard. You will be expected to help in-store promotions and, if you are interested and ambitious, might eventually aim for a job in marketing.

When an important new product is launched, the consultants are called into the head office to hear all about it and be instructed in its proper use. They may also be asked for their comments on current lines and customer reaction.

If you are good at your job, you may be promoted to demonstrator, with the job of travelling around the country giving public demonstrations on make-up and skin care in stores.

As a beauty consultant, you need to be extremely well groomed and have a pleasant and attractive manner. Consultants have to be an advertisement for the products that they are trying to sell, and being good at sales is an important part of the job. You should have a genuine interest in other people and be able to listen, hear what they say and be sympathetic to their problems. You should also have a good head for figures, as you will be involved with the counter-sales side of the work.

All the main cosmetics manufacturers run special short, intensive courses for beauty consultants, but these are not usually open to school-leavers. Rather, they are aimed at people in their early twenties who already have some selling experience. The minimum age for acceptance is age 18 and more mature entrants are preferred. If you are younger, it may be easier to find a job in the general cosmetics or perfumery department of a large store or chemist's shop, or to take a Saturday job while still studying. You will then become familiar with the range of goods available and learn how to deal with customers' queries. After some general experience in selling you can then apply to the cosmetics houses. It is probably best to write to the firms of your choice, who will then arrange to interview you. If you are accepted, you will be given several weeks on intensive training before being appointed to a store. To begin with, you will probably be working with an experienced consultant who knows what to do, but after a few months you are most likely to be working on your own.

The Hairdressing & Beauty Suppliers Organization (HBSA) does not offer any training but is an association of suppliers to the trade. Its Web site provides directories of suppliers and products as well as guides to relevant publications, events, exhibitions and seminars. The HBSA provides legal information, helplines for various aspects of the business, access to social events and trade show discounts. VTCT and ITEC offer training courses (see pages 78–79 for details).

Working freelance

If you work freelance, you have to have a thorough knowledge of all the major treatments. You will often be working alone in various situations and environments and will therefore have to be prepared to deal with the unexpected. You may market your services to clients who require home visits – the elderly, disabled or mothers with young children, and hospital and nursing homes will also require your services. A comprehensive range of quality equipment and products will be necessary to develop a portable salon. Proper maintenance of equipment is very important.

You will have to be self-motivated, well-organized and willing to travel. A car is essential. You should have NVQ/SVQ Level 2 and preferably NVQ/SVQ Level 3.

Trainer

If you want to go into full- or part-time teaching in the beauty industry you should have completed NVQ/SVQ Level 3. You will also have to take a further education Teacher's Certificate that can be gained in one or two years, as well as a PGCE.

Many combine part-time teaching with running a salon. Full-time teachers may spend about 20 hours per week teaching and around 10 hours in preparation, marking and assessment work. You will have to attend staff development courses to keep your skills and knowledge up to date with new developments.

Salon owner

As well as being very competent in your work, you will also need some management skills and business knowledge to run a successful salon. Self-motivation is essential and you must have strength of character as you will be working long hours, and perhaps after the salon has closed will have to deal with the administration, which includes book-keeping, PAYE and stock control. You must also recruit suitable staff. You will need a minimum NVQ/SVQ Level 3 but Level 4 is recommended.

Specialist places of work

Cruise liners

Working on a cruise liner involves all the practical beauty

therapy skills used in the day-to-day running of a salon. There is a special need for make-up artists as there are many formal evenings on board. As a cruise therapist, you will learn all aspects of business management and ship life, and training will include presentation, retail skills and customer service. You will be expected to sell beauty therapy services and products successfully to clients and should know about hairdressing treatments in order to promote the full range of services available. You will be part of a team where staff work together to serve a demanding clientele. You will have to be immaculately dressed, be able to get on with other people, and, of course, be willing to travel. The preferred qualification is NVQ/SVQ Level 3. Only fully qualified stylists will be considered for this specialist work.

Steiner Transocean Ltd is the leading spa operator worldwide and has spas on board over 100 cruise ships. There are many opportunities for beauty professional and nail technicians, with over 1,000 health and beauty experts being employed annually. With Steiner Training Ltd, new employees are trained up to Steiner's specific requirements, such as the use of certain specialist beauty treatments and the use of different products. Recruits will also have to learn microphone work for public speaking.

Luxury hotels

Many first-class hotels now offer health and beauty facilities. You will probably be dealing with an international, sophisticated and very demanding clientele who will be aware of the very latest treatments available and want very high standards of treatment. You will need to be both very fit and have the patience of a saint. The hours of work will vary according to demand. The work will be varied and interesting and the rates of pay good. The minimum qualifications recommended are NVQ/SVQ Level 3. Contact HABIA or BABTAC for further information.

In-flight beauticians/beauty therapists

This is a new concept that is proving very popular. The treatment is for first-class passengers who may receive manicures, pedicures, massage, to relieve tension and jet lag, and face treatments. You have to work well in a very confined space and be able to keep calm and cool under possibly very stressful conditions. You also have to radiate calm to what are probably nervous and anxious clients, who may also be difficult and demanding. In addition, you need to be able to mix well with the aircrew and avoid getting in their way. Recruitment is age 20–28 and you must have had some previous work experience in a salon.

Television and film industries

You must have completed a full-time course in beauty therapy or make-up and be at least aged 21 to be considered for training in this area of work. The first six months' training is spent learning the basic skills of TV make-up, and this is followed by six months on secondment to a hairdressing department. In the TV studio, make-up designers are responsible for research, design and the execution of make-up and hair for all productions. They also need to work closely with lighting directors and set designers as well as liaise with producers, directors, costume staff and artists. The hours worked are long and you will have to be willing to travel and live away from home for fairly long periods at a time. The competition for jobs is intense for the limited number of jobs available. To work in this area you will need a minimum of five GCSEs or equivalent and a minimum NVQ/SVQ Level 2 in beauty therapy, though Level 3 is preferred. You will also need to be creative and have a strong visual sense.

About 70 per cent of people working in the film and television industry are employed on short-term freelance contracts. It is desirable to have a driving licence and you should have good people and communication skills.

Further information from Film and Television Freelance Training, the BBC Corporation Recruitment Services and Skillset National Training Organization (NTO). (See pages 78 and 105 for training.)

Hospitals/care homes

Hospital salons cater for both patients and staff. Most hospitals and nursing homes use freelance beauticians or beauty therapists who will usually visit at prearranged times and on certain days of the week. It may be possible to use a designated room but more likely you will work in the patient's room. Health and safety regulations have to be strictly adhered to. You will have to work in difficult surroundings to make sure that you do not disrupt the patients, staff and visitors.

You have to be aware of the special needs of people in hospital and have a high degree of sympathy and understanding for your clients. The recommended NVQ/SVQ is Level 2 but Level 3 is preferred.

HM prison service

Beauticians or beauty therapists attend a one-week induction course covering prison policies, procedures and security arrangements within the prison. Some prisons offer the opportunity for inmates to train as beauty therapists or beauticians in preparation for employment when they return to the outside world, so there may be training posts available. Hours of work are normally Monday to Friday 8 am–4 pm. Stringent criteria are set for all personnel working in prisons and employees must be trustworthy and reliable. You will have to be especially tactful and be aware of your clients' special needs. A minimum NVQ/SVQ at Level 2 is required and Level 3 is preferred.

Leisure centres and health clubs

A number of mainly private leisure centres and health clubs have opportunities for staff in the beauty industry. This may include areas such as manicure, pedicure, facial scrubs, toning, massage, and aromatherapy. A minimum NVQ/SVQ at Level 2 is required.

Getting work in the beauty industry

Most people in the beauty industry work in salons. Unfortunately at present (2001) there is no regulation of beauty salons, either by law or on a voluntary basis. If you want to work in a particular salon, check it out very carefully before you apply for work. The room should be clean and the people should appear well groomed and busy. Ask your training organization or contact one of the organizations listed below for further advice.

Organizations connected with the beauty industry

◆ British Association of Beauty Therapy and Cosmetology (BABTAC) – An awarding body. CIDESCO's UK representative.
◆ Caribbean and Afro Society of Hairdressers – Specializes in African Caribbean hairdressing skills.
◆ Comité International d'Esthetique et de Cosmetologie (CIDESCO) – was founded in 1946 to establish international standards of professional ability and integrity in the beauty industry. It also aims to put members of the various countries in touch with each other for the exchange of professional knowledge and skills. CIDESCO training is available only at CIDESCO-approved beauty schools. There are over 140 CIDESCO schools worldwide and 80 accredited CIDESCO beauty centres.
◆ Confederation of International Beauty Therapy and Cosmetology (CIBTAC) – The examination body of BABTAC.
◆ Film and Television Freelance Training – A training organization for make-up artists.
◆ Guild of Professional Beauty Therapists – A leading organization for beauty therapy. Publishes a training directory and a magazine.
◆ Hairdressing and Beauty Industry Authority (HABIA) – The lead organization for beauty. Awards NVQs/SVQs in beauty therapy. Publishes a booklet, *Career Routes: the official guide to careers in hairdressing and beauty therapy.*

- Hairdressing and Beauty Suppliers Organization (HBSA) – Suppliers to the beauty industry.
- International Health and Beauty Council (IHBC) – A subsidiary of the VTCT. It runs over 20 courses in various fields of the beauty industry.
- Skillset – Subsidizes a range of short courses for freelancers in the beauty industry.
- Vocational Training Charitable Trust (VTCT) – Runs the NVQ/SVQ in Beauty Therapy at Levels 2 and 3 and in Customer Service at Levels 2 and 3. It also runs foundation and diploma courses in Anatomy and Physiology.

Fitness

There is a continuing interest in fitness as a method of promoting health and well-being. People of all ages are increasingly taking up fitness exercises, not only to keep in shape, reduce body fat and tone muscles but also to help improve their physical and mental condition. It is now accepted that being fit and in good health helps to increase an individual's ability to deal with stress and overcome depression.

There are currently (2001) over 3,500 privately owned and an additional 1,000 local authority fitness centres and clubs employing over 50,000 people and offering a very wide range of activities. The range includes large sports and leisure centres, which have hi-tech fitness suites and run fitness classes and aqua-aerobics and other pool-based exercise programmes; small private clubs, some within factories and offices, with pool facilities, sauna and a multi-gym; health studios offering fitness training for individuals and groups; the YMCA, offering all types of courses, and village halls, which run evening classes in aerobics, step, keep-fit and other exercise and movement instruction.

Types of work in the fitness industry

There are four main types of work. In small clubs the functions can often be combined, with staff having to be able to turn their hands to anything that is required to run the centre. In larger clubs, however, there are usually managers and staff who work in separate spheres only such as the gym, swimming, spa pool, reception, administration and food and drinks departments.

Receptionists/sales personnel

There are now people in the fitness industry who work only in the sales and marketing departments of clubs and who control membership admin. If you want to work in this area you will not need to be fully trained in fitness and exercise techniques but you will need to have good interpersonal skills and sales training. IT skills are also important. Many sales staff travel to visit local companies to give presentations and work with local journalists and reporters.

There are no specific qualifications required but it is a good idea to aim for the NVQ/SVQ Level 1 in Sport, Recreation and Allied Occupations (see page 83) or the BTEC HNC in Leisure Management, Sport and Recreation and Outdoor Activities (see page 86).

Recreation assistants

Recreation assistants have to make sure the environment and the equipment used is safe for use by the clients. You have to deal with risk assessment, hazard management and ensure that all equipment is in good working condition. You also have to be responsible for the cleanliness of the building and see that standards of safety, environmental control and hygiene are maintained during working hours.

Relevant qualifications include the BTEC HNC in Leisure Management, Sport and Recreation and Outdoor Activities (see page 86) or the ISRM Sport and Recreation Management Certificate (see page 89).

Fitness instructor

There are many activities that fitness instructors may specialize in and teach to individuals and/or groups. For instance, there is aerobics, an overall body exercise, which increases oxygen levels in the blood, often delivered as an hour-long exercise to music.

'Step' involves participants working around a small step or plat-form. 'Slide' involves lateral motion exercise to improve aerobic fitness and muscular condition. 'Weight' in the fitness room mostly refers to exercise machines and fixed and variable resis-tance apparatus and using free weights. There is also circuit training for which instructors devise programmes aimed at developing overall fitness for the whole body. Participants complete different exercises at a number of exercise stations with rest time between each station. Another area is exercise in water and there are an increasing number of pool-based exer-cise classes. It is not just a straight transfer of dry exercise to the pool; when designing an aqua exercise programme, instructors have to take account of buoyancy, resistance and how water affects both balance and movement.

If you are a fitness instructor working in a gym, you will have to supervise clients and make sure they are exercising safely and effectively. You will write personalized programmes and super-vise and demonstrate the use of equipment as well as carry out medical screening and inductions, and sometimes take group exercise classes such as aerobics or circuit training.

In many centres, related services are available to clients, for example, sunbeds and toning tables, which provide passive exer-cise. As a fitness instructor, you will be on hand to give advice about the whole range of equipment on offer.

If you are highly experienced and more qualified you may do one-to-one work with clients, called personal training. You may then be known as a fitness practitioner.

You need to be very fit and healthy. You also need to be confident and have an interest in people and have a real desire to help them, with a relaxed manner. You need to be able to encourage and motivate people and to explain things in a straightforward way. People going to a class or fitness club for the first time may be very shy and self-conscious (especially if seriously overweight or out of condition), and it will be your job to put them at ease and help them to relax and enjoy the exercises. If what they do is too painful, exhausting or humili-ating, your clients are unlikely to come back for more. Instructing demands patience and you will have to assess your clients' capabilities and pace exercise programmes accordingly.

You may have to adapt certain exercises to suit people's needs, perhaps taking into account an individual's health or injury problems. You will also have to recognize when a client has a serious health problem and should be referred to a doctor.

Most instructors will receive vocational training as well as specific training leading to an industry-recognized qualification such as the NVQ/SVQ Level 2 in one area of the Sport, Recreation and Allied Occupations (see pages 83–85). You are also strongly advised to take an ITEC course relating to fitness instruction (see pages 87–88).

Case Study

John *is a fitness instructor in a sports centre.*

'I didn't really know what I wanted to do at 16, but I was interested in sport so decided to take a one-year full-time City & Guilds course in Recreation and Leisure. At the end of the year, the college introduced a two-year BTEC National Diploma and this led to doing a BTEC HND in Leisure Management at Carnegie College in Leeds. I converted the HND to a BSc (Hons) by doing an extra year. These full-time courses have been very useful, but really for anyone interested in a career in this field study alone is not enough. My part-time work experience has helped a lot – I have worked weekends and holidays as a leisure assistant and lifeguard at the Metrodome (the main sports and leisure centre) for the last six years. As far as I am concerned the RLSS (Royal Lifesaving Saving Society) bronze award is essential – so many fitness centres, even the small private clubs, have swimming pools. Your chances of employment are far greater if you can offer a number of skills. I don't think this is emphasized enough at college.

'I've just started here as the fitness instructor and I am continuing to do weekends at the Metrodome for the time being. When customers first come here, I take them through an induction where I introduce them to all the equipment. They have a go and I make an initial assessment of their abilities. An individual fitness programme is worked out for every client. A programme begins with a warm-up on the cardiovascular equipment – steppers, joggers and bikes – then moves on to the resistance training machines, starting off with equipment for large muscles such as shoulders, chest and back, then works on the smaller muscle groups.

'Everyone fills in a record card when they first come here. It contains relevant medical information as well as personal details such as weight, height and fitness levels. When devising a programme, I consider this information, along with people's aims. For instance, body fat reduction or strength development. The programme tells the client what weights to put on to the different machines and how many exercises to do. I give instruction on how to use equipment safely and give advice, for example, on stretching exercises before using the resistance machines. After a few sessions I might adapt a programme, say, if it is too easy or too hard, and I will revise programmes as people progress. I don't make programmes too difficult; this is with safety in mind and also so that clients will enjoy their exercise and come back for more. It might be beneficial for someone to work on a particular machine but if they don't like the machine there is no point in pushing it. Often people come round to wanting to try out such machines once they begin to feel the benefits of being fit.

'My hours are 1–9 pm, but I have to put in more to do the job well. Last night I stayed until 9.30 and then worked at home on fitness programmes until 1 am. Long, unsociable hours are a fact of life with jobs in the leisure industry, so that's something you've got to be prepared for. Rates of pay can be quite low, too, especially at first. Another aspect of this work is that training is an ongoing process. I'm going to take the Institute of Sports and Recreation Management qualifications, which will help with my long-term goals of leisure centre management. My advice to anyone thinking about a career in this field is to take all the opportunities for experience and training that you can – employers are looking for commitment.'

Case Study

Kathleen *is a qualified RSA Exercise to Music Teacher.*

'I have always been interested in exercise, from being involved in athletics at school. I decided that I wanted to get into fitness in a big way and make it part of a career for myself. I wanted to do aerobics so enrolled at the local college to do the RSA Basic Certificate in the Teaching of Exercise to Music course. The course is normally two classes a week for around six months, although I had extra tuition once a week as I felt I needed it, having been away from education for a relatively long time. Two or three times a week I participated in aerobics classes to maintain and improve my own fitness, which is so important.

'It is amazing how quickly aerobics can improve your fitness level. When I first began, I considered myself as fairly unfit, but that soon changed. It is not just a matter of physical fitness and speeding up your reactions; with aerobics all your systems, nervous systems, cardiovascular systems and so on, become fitter so it helps with mental health and being able to handle situations in everyday life.

'After qualifying, I set about running an aerobics class. First, I found out where there was a suitable hall and arranged to hire it for two evenings a week. The other practical aspects were organizing the necessary insurance, buying workout mats and advertising the classes – I put up some hand-written posters locally and managed to get the local paper interested in doing a feature on me for their 'People's Page'. The other thing is the music; you can't just make your own tapes because copyright legislation affects the public use of sound recordings. What I do is buy tapes that carry a licence. There are a number of companies that supply the tapes, specifically designed for use in aerobics and exercise.

'I plan my classes to incorporate the main components of aerobic exercise starting with mobility exercises: mobilizing all the joints for free movement. We move on to a pulse raiser to get the body warm, ready to pre-stretch all the muscles before going into the aerobics. The aerobics itself has three components: the build-up, gradually bringing the pulse up, the peak when the heart and lungs are really working, and then the cool-down where big movements are gradually converted into small movements and the pace is slowed down. After the aerobics we move on to muscular strength exercises, then relaxation. I end with a remobilizer – either something funny or a co-ordination test – to make people feel uplifted when they leave.

'I try to bring the class to the level of the participants; if a class is too hard, people won't come back. I also try to make my classes fun, again so that people will come back. Planning the class involves choosing appropriate music for the different stages. I work out what should fit into an hour, but obviously have to adapt this during the class. One of the most important parts of the job is watching the participants carefully. It is essential to correct people if they are not exercising properly, so you have to make sure the exercise is effective and, most importantly, that the participants don't hurt themselves.

'I really love teaching, even more than participating. There is a remarkable sense of achievement when everything comes together and flows nicely. It is wonderful to feel that I've taught a safe and effective class.'

Club manager

This is a demanding position with responsibility for the day-to-day working of the club or centre. It requires a high level of management skill, financial control and customer relations. You will need to prepare progress reports for the owner or operator and will need to be computer-literate. You will need at least seven years experience in the fitness industry, a good academic qualification and specialist training.

If you want to be a club manager you are strongly advised to take either the ISRM Supervisory Management Certificate or the Sport and Recreation Management Certificate (see pages 88–89).

Specialist fitness organizations

The Fitness League's system aims to achieve and maintain good posture as well as easy, relaxed and harmonious body movement. Exercises are carried out to music, which is carefully selected to assist the pace and rhythm of the exercises. Members' ages range from 6 to 80. There are two stages to becoming a teacher: Stage 1 involves 98 contact hours and attendance at Fitness League classes; Stage 2 is in modular form and comprises six credits of 12 hours each.

The Keep Fit Association (KFA) offers fitness through dance, movement and exercise. It is an awarding body for movement and dance/dance fitness. In addition to improving stamina, strength and suppleness, the KFA offers improved movement skills in balance, agility and co-ordination.

The Medau approach is one of whole body natural movement, with emphasis on using the body correctly. Medau emphasizes good posture and body alignment in various exercises run to music.

The Margaret Morris Movement is a form of dance and exercise, particularly suited for people with disabilities. It has 11 grades, offering the opportunity for anyone to work through the initial co-ordinated exercises, providing the basic requirements of strength, control and body awareness to enable the individual to move on to higher grades of pure dance if desired.

Getting work in the fitness industry

Check with your training college about vacancies, or look for vacancies in specialist magazines or journals, such as *Health Club Management* and *Leisure Manager, Leisureweek* and *BodyLife UK*. You might have a friend who knows of a vacancy. Phone some of the organizations connected with the fitness industry listed below for further information. You might want to try contacting a fitness recruitment agency such as Fitness Recruitment Ltd or the Web site www.alive2000.com that focus on health and fitness. SPRITO has published a guide for students on how to get into the field (see page 115). Work is not difficult to find because the industry is expanding very fast.

Organizations connected with the fitness industry

◆ The British Association of Sport and Exercise Sciences (BASES) – BASES aims to develop and spread knowledge about the application of science to sport and exercise.
◆ Fitness Industry Association – An employer/trade association for operators of health and fitness clubs. It works proactively to promote best practice.
◆ Fitness League – Provides a comprehensive teacher training course.
◆ Fitness Northern Ireland – The governing body for fitness and exercise in Northern Ireland. Organizes courses and workshops.
◆ Fitness Professionals (FitPro) – A professional organization for fitness instructors and personal trainers.
◆ Fitness Recruitment Ltd – Has lists of job vacancies available on a Web site.
◆ Fitness Scotland – The governing body for fitness and exercise in Scotland. Provides courses in exercise to music, step, circuit and gym. A new dance fitness course is available from 2001.
◆ Fitness Wales – The governing body for fitness and exercise in Wales. Organizes various fitness instructor courses.
◆ Institute of Sport and Recreation Management (ISRM) – Aims to improve the management and operation of sport and recreation services in communities through the provision of standard setting, training, information and consultancy services.
◆ Keep Fit Association (KFA) – Offers fitness through dance, movement and exercise. An awarding body.

- Margaret Morris Movement – Training courses in dance and movement available. Courses for teachers are run country-wide.
- Medau Movement – Has a teacher training course in the Medau movement.
- National Training Organization for Sport, Recreation and Allied Occupations (SPRITO) – Developed the national standards upon which the NVQs related to fitness are based.
- Sports Coach UK – Sports Coach UK offers a wide range of workshops at a number of different levels in fitness and training.
- Steiner Transocean – Trains and recruits aerobics and fitness instructors for cruise ships.
- YMCA Fitness Industry Training – Provides fitness training courses.

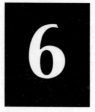

6 Fitness therapies

The following six therapies normally come under the heading of alternative medicine. They are, however, actually nothing to do with medicine and fit much better under the category of fitness therapies. They teach methods of keeping fit and aim to promote good health. Fitness therapies are rapidly expanding and job prospects are very good. It is very important, however, to receive proper training. As the various techniques listed are unregulated, this means that anyone can set up as a therapist, even those with hardly any training. For details of good quality training, contact the umbrella organizations listed after each therapy for further details.

Alexander Technique

The Alexander Technique teaches new ways of thinking about and using our bodies so we can eliminate unconscious habits of tension, particularly those that constrict the spine, thereby improving physical and psychological well-being. Primarily, the Technique aims to remove the cause, not the symptoms, of disorders. Practitioners see the Technique as a way of living rather than as a therapy, and as a method of promoting well-being through psychophysical re-education rather than as treating dysfunction. A fundamental principle of the Technique is that the mind and body are interconnected and interact with each other. Teachers of the Technique do not profess to treat or claim to cure anything. They refer to themselves as teachers and those who come to them as pupils. Pupils are taught to become aware of balance, posture and movement as applied to all actions in everyday life, such as thinking, breathing, eating, speaking, walking, reading and lying down.

Case Study

Hilary *teaches the Alexander Technique at various centres, as well as privately, in London.*

'Initially I trained in ballet and, while doing this, strained my back. I heard about the Alexander Technique through some musicians. Later I did a psychology degree at a college and found it a great strain doing the exams. My mother died of a heart attack and I thought I would end up like her if I wasn't careful. There was a lecturer who also taught the Alexander Technique at the college and I initially learnt the Technique from him. It helped me to sort out my old back injury and to cope with high stress levels.

'I trained as a teacher at the North London Teacher Training Centre, which I thought was excellent – very warm and caring. Those who taught me had an excellent understanding of the Technique and how to use it. The school's atmosphere was good, which is very important as it enables the students to have the courage to make changes in them-selves. There were also a lot of visiting teachers, some of whom gave talks as well as taking part in class activities.

'I see approximately 20 to 25 people a week. My lessons are either half an hour or 40 minutes each, on a one-to-one basis. I devote half the lesson doing simple activities like sitting, standing or walking around while I guide pupils into improving their psychophysical use. The other half is devoted to a lying-down procedure on a table. Pupils learn to develop awareness and learn how to give themselves directions to help themselves. We learn to recognize how, where and why we create patterns of tension and misuse, in response to thoughts, emotions and external stimuli, and how to inhibit and stop habitual patterns of behav-iour. Lessons are a process of exploration and discovery. A teacher's hands and verbal instructions guide pupils through activities such as sitting and standing; in that way their misuse may be recognized and a new way of being may be experienced. Once pupils learn to recognize, understand and then inhibit their patterns of misuse, they are freer to choose new and more effective physical and mental responses to situa-tions, while at the same time gaining more awareness, poise and co-ordination.

'I like working with people and find the work very positive and creative. I enjoy helping people to use themselves in a freer manner; it's really rewarding when people's problems or performance levels improve. Also, I find it really positive to have to work on myself at the same time as I work on my pupils.'

Further information from the Society of Teachers of the Alexander Technique (see page 91 for training details).

Feldenkrais

The Feldenkrais method teaches people to move easily with minimum effort and maximum efficiency. It helps to improve balance and co-ordination and to alleviate back and neck pain, clumsiness, stiffness, stress and other musculoskeletal or neurological problems and poor self-image. It improves digestion, sleep patterns, alertness and flexibility. The method positively affects a person's physical, emotional and mental well-being. Further information from the Feldenkrais Guild UK and Feldenkrais International Training Centre Ltd (see pages 91–92 for training details).

Massage

Massage, using stroking and kneading techniques, relaxes and revives the body and mind physically, mentally and emotionally. Today in the West there are around 100 different types of massage, which is often used in conjunction with other therapies, particularly aromatherapy (see page 17).

Various forms of touch are applied to the muscles and ligaments of the body and are designed to relax, strengthen and stimulate. Massage helps to relieve pain, free and mobilize stiff joints and aids recovery from minor soft tissue problems. It also enables the digestive system to function efficiently, and it is known to ease tensions and knotted tissue, increase the circulation of the blood and stimulate the lymphatic system which helps to eliminate waste material. Further information from The British Federation of Massage Practitioners or the British Massage Therapy Council (see page 92 for training details).

Pilates

Pilates is a body-conditioning programme comprising eight main principles: relaxation, co-ordination, alignment, concentration, flowing movements, centring, breathing and stamina. The method aims to re-align and re-balance the body's structure through gentle but focused exercise, to improve posture and to increase flexibility and strength without building bulk muscle. It helps those with bad backs or general injuries and is excellent for rehabilitation after surgery. It is also a good form of exercise both during and after surgery. Futher information from the Pilates Foundation (see pages 92–93 for training details).

T'ai chi ch'uan

T'ai chi ch'uan, usually shortened to t'ai chi, is a Chinese martial art. It was originally employed for the purpose of self-defence but is now used for health and spiritual development. It is also used as a therapy for the prevention and treatment of disease. You learn how to think and move in ways governed by principles and methods of practice, and are taught to become aware of the natural laws that govern change. There are six main t'ai chi principles. You are taught to relax both your mind and body, in order to discover your inner strength and become centred and focused. You are also shown how important it is to concentrate, to keep the mind connected to what your body is experiencing. You are taught how to enable the body and mind to respond spontaneously to immediate needs of the moment. Through the exercises, you are shown how to be consistent in your thoughts and actions, so that you can achieve your goals. You are also taught to value slow but steady progress and, if necessary, to delay the gratification of achievement, to allow time to gain what you want. The final principle, which perhaps is the most difficult to achieve, is to learn to accept life's challenges.

For further information about t'ai chi, look at the Web site www.taichi-online.com – also, you can contact the British

Council for Chinese Martial Arts. This is the UK governing body, recognized by the Sports Council, and represents over 10,000 members across all of the major disciplines of Chinese martial arts. The Tai Chi Union is highly recommended and has the largest collective of independent t'ai chi instructors in the British Isles. It exists to unite t'ai chi practitioners, promote t'ai chi in all its aspects, including health, aesthetic meditation and self-defence and to improve standards and collate and disseminate information on t'ai chi classes. Also highly recommended are Practical Tai Chi Chuan, T'ai Chi UK and Herts Long Fei Taijiquan Association. (See pages 110–11.)

Yoga

There are many different kinds of yoga. The method that has been taken up in the West is hatha yoga, from the Sanskrit 'ha' meaning 'sun' and 'tha', 'moon', implying balance. Hatha yoga is the physical expression of yogic practices demonstrated through physical postures. It is a holistic approach to self-development and a means of self-help towards physical and mental health.

There are no set patterns of teaching hatha yoga and ideally, a yoga teacher should tailor routines to suit each individual. The aim is to integrate the mind and body. Physical postures known as *asanas* may be performed by either standing, kneeling, sitting or lying on your back or front. There are regular intervals when deep relaxation exercises are taught as well as controlled breathing exercises known as *pranayama*.

Traditionally, a guru (teacher) teaches yoga to disciples. Yoga classes differ widely and there is no one institution that supervises teachers. The training needed to qualify as a yoga teacher may vary from a few weeks to two or three years, preceded by several years of regular practice. Yoga postures and breathing are effective only if practised regularly. Practice is a major requirement for teachers who should also have knowledge of anatomy and physiology as well as a thorough training in their own particular branch of yoga. Further information from the British School of Yoga, the British Wheel of Yoga or the Iyengar Yoga Institute (see pages 93–94 for training details).

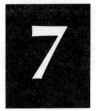

7 Getting started and finding a job

Having made the decision to work in the hairdressing, beauty or fitness industries, what do you do next? Before you do anything else, think hard about your decision. Have you really decided to go for it? A golden rule to remember is that you have to really want to do something before you can do it. A half-baked attempt to find a job will lead nowhere. But, if you are determined, sure you want the job and are focused on what you are doing, you will get what you want.

Once you are sure that you want to go ahead, you can set about finding a job.

Finding a job

There are very many different ways of finding jobs. You can, for instance, ask for news of jobs at your training college, go to an agency, check specialist newspapers that carry advertisements or go directly to a salon or health or fitness club.

You might want to apply direct to a salon or club to find out if there are any vacancies. You could just walk in on a quiet day (say, Monday or Tuesday) and ask to speak to the manager, who will give you the information you require about vacancies, hours of work, salaries and benefits. If there is a definite vacancy, the manager may say whether he or she considers the job suitable for you and may help you to decide whether you definitely want to apply for it.

If you find the idea of walking into a salon or club a bit daunting, you could always write a letter or telephone. If you phone, ask for an application form for the job, or, if there isn't one available, ask for an interview. Go straight to the point and say something like: 'I'm ringing about the job advertised in today's paper/on the television/on the Internet, in the window. It sounds interesting. Could you tell me more about it, please?' You may be asked for an interview on the phone there and then, so do be prepared (see 'Telephone interviews' below). If you are writing a letter, ask whether there are vacancies of the type you require, if you don't know already, and for further information and an application form.

On a *separate sheet of paper*, give some *brief* details about your age, where you were educated and your qualifications. This is called your curriculum vitae (CV for short), and the way this is set out is shown below.

You may have a friend or relative who knows of an available job and who is willing to help you. Perhaps he or she already works in the salon or club you want to work in, in which case you can learn about the people you might be going to work with, what sort of money you are likely to earn, what the building is like and, most important, the way the staff are treated by their boss.

Listen to what your friend or relative has to say. If what is said sounds attractive, then you can apply feeling confident that at least one person likes working for the salon or club you are considering. If, on the other hand, the prospects sound gloomy, you can decide either to forget the whole thing, or apply anyway, on the basis that there might be a good job for you, even though the person giving you the information is unhappy. It just might be that you know he or she is liable to moan about most things. So ignore the gloomy side, pick out the good bits, and decide, if you are asked to attend an interview, to judge for yourself.

The letter of application and application form

If you are phoning the salon or club you want to work in, you may well be asked to attend an interview immediately, or possibly have an interview over the phone. If, however, you are applying for a job through the post you will have to write a letter of application for the job. You should be very careful about this letter. *Keep it short and to the point.* Mention where you saw the advertisement for the vacancy you are applying for (if there is a definite vacancy) and keep a copy of the letter for reference. The person receiving it will not want a torn or dirty bit of paper, full of words that are difficult to read because they are misspelt, or a letter written in scrawly writing. It is vital you check your spelling in a draft letter.

Once you have written and checked the draft letter, write it out again, very neatly and send it off with a first-class stamp. If you are typing the letter, use the spell-check on your computer's word-processing system.

After you have sent an initial letter, you may receive an application form. Application forms are carefully designed and ask for personal details about your education, job experience, and other activities and interests. You should fill in the form, answering all the questions asked, and keep your answers as short as possible – unless asked to do otherwise.

The curriculum vitae

You may be asked to send in a curriculum vitae (CV), if you haven't already done so. This is a summary of your life to date, with details of your educational background, qualifications and work experience. It should be typed, if possible, and should not be more than two pages long. It should give the following details:

- full name and address;
- date of birth;
- schools attended;
- examinations passed;
- any other honours won at school;
- any particular position of authority held at school;
- training courses or colleges attended and qualifications gained;

- previous jobs held or any other experience gained, including details of any work experience such as holiday or Saturday jobs;
- present employment, if any;
- personal interests or hobbies;
- mention current driving licence, if you have one;
- names, addresses and phone numbers of two referees – one of these should be a previous employer, if you have had one, or someone who has personal knowledge of your capabilities.

Telephone interviews

There is an increasing trend, particularly in the hairdressing and beauty industries, towards initial interviewing by phone. If the employer likes the sound of you during a preliminary phone interview, you will probably be asked to come along later for a more formal interview. As the phone interview may take place immediately you apply for the job, it is important you are well prepared. Bear in mind the following:

- Write out all the relevant details about yourself on a piece of paper in case you get flustered (see the details for the CV required above).
- Before you first speak, take a deep breath and try not to gabble with nerves. Try to speak in a firm, clear voice. Don't mumble, and try to cut out as many 'ums', 'ers', 'sort ofs' and 'you knows' as possible. Remember that your voice is the only thing the employer has to go on, so even if you don't feel confident you must try to sound pleasant, self-assured and capable.
- It is best to use a phone where you know you are not going to be interrupted by other people. If you have to ring from a payphone, make sure you have an ample supply of coins, or buy a Phonecard and make sure you can use a Phonecard telephone. Don't use a mobile phone as it is sure to lose reception at a very awkward moment.

Face-to-face interviews

You will almost certainly be asked for a face-to-face interview before starting a new job. You may feel nervous about this – almost everyone does, no matter how many interviews they have been through. Remember that for most jobs your appearance and manner will be considered almost as important as your general level of education and diplomas. Bear in mind the following checklist of points to remember:

♦ Be on time for the interview. If you are even two minutes late, this will count against you, so leave for the interview in plenty of time, allowing for traffic jams, late trains, tube hold-ups, etc.

♦ Be well groomed, with clean clothes and shoes, clean hands and nails and tidy hair. If you are a man, make sure your shirt does not hang out of your trousers and if a woman wearing trousers, make sure they are smart. Dress neatly rather than flashily. Whatever you wear should be clean and well pressed.

♦ Smile pleasantly, look directly at the interviewer, and try to make eye contact.

♦ Don't smoke even if invited to do so.

♦ Speak clearly without mumbling. Your tone of voice will be a very important consideration for the interviewer. Don't giggle or make jokey remarks. Try to avoid giving 'yes' and 'no' answers, but on the other hand, don't ramble on.

♦ Don't allow yourself to get angry or irritated at anything the interviewer says. He or she may be finding out how well you stand up to pressure. Try to keep cool and unfazed, no matter how the conversation goes.

♦ Be honest about what you perceive your abilities to be, but at the same time remember that you have to sell yourself to your prospective employer. Talk about your good points and what you can do, rather than what you can't do.

♦ Above all, try to appear interested in the job. An employer will always prefer someone who seems lively and enthusiastic.

You may find interviews less frightening if you remember that there is always a structure. The interviewer will probably start by putting you at your ease, making small talk about the weather or your journey to the interview. He or she will then fairly quickly move on to try to draw you out by asking about your career to date and what you have been doing since you left school. The interviewer will want you to talk to get an impression of your manner with people. Then your letter of application and CV will be discussed in detail. It is important at this point not to show that you are bored or irritated. Everything being asked may already be there on paper, but be prepared to give the details again, politely.

Make sure you have an answer ready when you are asked how you see your career developing, or what you would like to be doing in five years' time. Also, be ready for the question 'Why are you applying for this particular job?' Even if you have been sent by an agency, you must still make it sound as if *you* are keen on the job and want to apply for it. The interviewer will probably then ask if you have a clear picture of the job and what it entails. This is to find out if you have really thought about what you might be doing.

At the end of the interview, the interviewer will probably ask if you have any questions, and you must try to think of something to say. If it looks as if you are going to be offered the job, this is the moment when you can clear up anything you are not sure about. You could, for example, ask how your training will be organized or how many weeks' holiday you are entitled to. The interviewer will be pleased you have asked these questions as it will be obvious you are showing real interest in the job and that you are well motivated.

Finally, you should ask to see round the place where you might be working so that you can get a good look at it and perhaps meet some of the people you might be working with.

Accepting a job

Before you write your official letter of acceptance, you should make sure you know exactly where you stand. You should know the sort of things you are going to be expected to do in the job, what your hours and rates of pay are, and how many week's holiday you get per year. You should make sure you know all these things *before* you accept the job offer. It is no use saying that you didn't realize what the job involved, or that you thought you were entitled to five weeks' holiday and it turns out to be only four, after you have accepted the job and are already working in your place of employment.

Contract of employment

A contract of employment exists as soon as someone offers you a job, even verbally, at a certain rate of pay, and you accept. Within two months of you starting work, whether full-time or part-time, the employer is required by law to give you written particulars of certain key terms of your contract. These cover the following:

- names of employer and employee;
- date when employment began;
- expected period of employment or date of termination if employment is temporary or for a fixed term;
- job title and job description;
- place of work, or whether you are required to work in various locations;
- pay;
- sickness or injury and sick pay;
- how you are paid (whether weekly, monthly, etc);
- hours of work;
- holiday entitlement and pay;
- length of notice required;
- disciplinary and grievance procedures;
- pension rights;
- collective agreements.

If you are not given these particulars within two months of starting work, you should ask for them. All documents that you receive from your employer are important, and may comprise part of your contract of employment, so make sure you keep them in a safe place.

Your contract may be subject to your employer receiving satisfactory references. You may also be placed on an initial probationary period for the first few months to assess your suitability. During such a period, you may not enjoy the same level of benefits as your colleagues in permanent positions. If your employer is not fully satisfied with your performance he or she may dismiss you during or at the end of your probationary period or may extend the period of probation.

Career development loans

These are loans ranging from £300–£8,000 to individuals to support vocational training courses lasting up to two years and, if relevant, for up to one year's practical work experience where it forms part of the course. Courses can be full-time, part-time or distance learning courses. Applicants can be employed, self-employed or unemployed.

Career Development Loans are commercial loans offered through four high street banks. The DfES pays interest on the loan for the length of the course and up to one month afterwards. Applicants who are unemployed, or in work and in receipt of certain state benefits, on completion of their course may apply to have the repayment period deferred for up to a further 18 months. Further information from the DfES: 0800 585505 or www.dfes.gov.uk.

Employment Service Direct

Employment Service Direct is a phone service set up to help you find a full- or part-time job. Help can be obtained from qualified staff to find the most suitable vacancies for you. Telephone advisers have immediate access to all the jobs that might be suitable for you. They can send job application forms or arrange interviews over the phone. The lines are open Mon–Fri 9 am–6 pm and Saturdays 9 am–1 pm. For further information, phone 0845 6060234 (textphone 0845 6055255).

New Deal

New Deal started in April 1998, and was created to help people find lasting, worthwhile work. It is mainly for people aged 18–24 who have been unemployed for six months or more and who are claiming Jobseeker's Allowance. The scheme offers individual tailored practical help and support to improve a person's job prospects and to build up the skills needed by local businesses.

If you join the New Deal scheme, you will begin with a period of concentrated individual help lasting for up to four months. You will receive a weekly subsidy for up to six months and employers will receive help towards the cost of providing training of one day a week (or equivalent) towards an approved qualification. There is a strong emphasis on meeting basic skill needs, which will normally lead to an NVQ/SVQ Level 2. For further information, contact www.newdeal.gov.uk.

Part-time working

Part-time workers now have the same employment protection rights as full-time workers, regardless of the number of hours they work per week. For example, both part-time and full-time workers have the right not to be unfairly dismissed and the right to a redundancy payment provided they have worked for the same employer for at least two years.

Working Time Regulations

Working Time Regulations (WTR) came into force on 1 October 1998. The basic rights and protections that the WTR provides are as follows:

♦ a limit of an average of 48 hours a week that a worker can be required to work (though workers can choose to work more if they want to);

- a limit of an average of 8 hours work in 24 that night-workers can be required to work;
- a right for night-workers to receive free health assessments;
- a right to 11 hours rest a day;
- a right to an in-work rest break if the working day is longer than six hours;
- a right to four weeks' paid leave per year.

The entitlements, that is, for example, the rest periods, breaks and annual leave are enforced through employment tribunals, although ACAS will initially endeavour to resolve any dispute. The working time limits are enforced by the Health and Safety Executive (HSE) and local authorities. Further information from the HSE enquiry line: 08701 545500.

Equal opportunities

Your employer should have implemented an equal opportunities policy to ensure the recruitment process and workplace are free from discrimination on the grounds of sex, race or disability.

Sex or racial discrimination may occur either where a person is treated less favourably because of his or her sex or race (direct discrimination), or where an employer imposes an unjustifiable condition that you are unable to satisfy because of your sex or race (indirect discrimination).

Disability discrimination occurs where a person is unjustifiably disadvantaged because of a disability. Your employer may be required to make reasonable adjustments to the workplace or recruitment process to prevent discrimination. For these purposes, a disability is a physical or mental impairment that has a substantial and long-term adverse affect on a person's ability to carry out normal day-to-day activities.

Flexible working patterns

There is a growing trend for flexible working patterns. This means that you can be employed to work a certain number of hours per week, but that, when you work, those hours will vary from week to week. Employers in such circumstances require flexibility from their employees and you should find out before you accept a job what hours you will be expected to work to ensure that you can fulfil the employer's requirements or that you will be guaranteed a minimum number of working hours.

Minimum wage rates

The National Minimum Wage Act became law on 1 April 1999 to enforce a statutory minimum wage, making it illegal for employers to pay less. The Act applies to employers in the UK. The standard minimum wage as from 1 October 2001 is £4.10, with a youth rate for 18–21 year olds of £3.50. Full-time and part-time workers are covered by the Act as are freelance workers, but workers under the age of 18 and apprentices and undergraduates on sandwich courses are not covered. There is also an accredited training rate at a minimum wage of £3.20 per hour and is for workers aged 22 and over who start a new job with a new employer and do accredited training. Accredited training is a course approved by the UK government to obtain a vocational qualification. The rate can only be paid for the first six months of the new job, after which the worker must get at least £4.10 an hour.

Further information from www.tiger.gov.uk or the National Minimum Wage helpline on 0845 6000 678. The helpline opening hours are Mon–Fri 8 am–6 pm.

8 Top Tips for getting in and getting on

♦ Work on a voluntary basis or take on some part-time work before you apply for a 'proper' job. That way you can find out if you like the work and, if you do, you will be able to say that you've had some valuable work experience later, when you go for an interview. You will show you are both willing and keen to work and you will have gained useful experience of dealing with clients. In any event, you will be learning on the job, both how to do it right and, most important, how not to make mistakes!

♦ Keep an eye on the local, national and specialist newspapers, magazines and journals for jobs advertised.

♦ Check out your local salons for work in hairdressing and beauty.

♦ Keep abreast of current trends. Read up on your chosen topic, whether it is fashion or keep-fit magazines or journals. Any knowledge you acquire will help to make you a better informed, more useful member of the organization you want to enter.

♦ Keep fit! If you want to be a fitness instructor or personal trainer you will have to be 100 per cent fit all the time, but even if you want to work in a salon as a hairdresser, beauty therapist or make-up artist you have to be fitter than most. You will be on your feet for almost all of the day and constantly moving about. Also, if you work freelance you will be lugging your equipment around with you. To keep fit, make sure you get enough sleep each night and that you sleep well. Eat sensibly: lots of fruit and vegetables, a little meat and fish (unless you're vegetarian) and only a few cakes, sweets and puddings. Drink lots of water and not too much alcohol. If you smoke, give it up, otherwise you'll start huffing and puffing and coughing. Do make sure you get plenty of fresh air. Try to go for a short, brisk walk in your lunch break.

◆ Don't be late. Time-keeping is very important in your work. You don't want to turn up late and find an irate client. When you go for an interview it is, of course, essential you turn up at the time agreed.

◆ Look neat, tidy and well groomed. As a hairdresser or someone working in the beauty world, you will have to look rather better than your clients so that you give a good impression. Even as a fitness trainer you will give a bad impression if your hair is unkempt and straggly, or your clothes look ruffled and ragged. Remember that you are always on display so you must look the part.

◆ Self-motivation is very important. Take the initiative and don't rely on others to do your thinking for you. Organize your work carefully. Read up on the latest trends, and practise them. Suggest new features for your place of work.

◆ Look alert, look interested and try to smile. Your clients are not going to like it if you appear listless, bored and grumpy. You have to show you want to be with people and that you are interested in hearing what they have to say. A pleasing face with a smile shows a likeable person who fits in with other people.

The future of the hairdressing, beauty and fitness industries

In 2001, hairdressing, beauty and fitness are forecast to be growth industries. In the UK and Republic of Ireland people are becoming ever more concerned with their image, and youth culture predominates. Therefore an increasing number of older people are seeking to look younger and fitter. It is not, however, only older people who want to look good and feel fit. Increasing demands are made upon people's time in the modern world, which means that time has become more scarce and precious. People are buying time in ways that would have been considered inconceivable even 20 years ago. Instead of doing your hair yourself, you get it done for you; instead of making yourself look good, you get someone else to do this. With the ever-increasing demand for the services of these industries, there will be a greater number of hairdressing and beauty salons and fitness and health centres provided. This means, of course, that more staff will be required.

With the greater awareness of the need to keep fit to live longer and more comfortably, the fitness industry is increasing very rapidly. A further 600–1,000 fitness centres and clubs are expected to open within the next few years and it is estimated that the industry will grow by 50 per cent over the next five years, that is, by over 8 per cent a year. So, opportunities for work in the fitness industry are very good. Currently, a number of studies are taking place to ensure better regimes and see how fitness can be achieved in the shortest time possible. This will undoubtedly mean that even within the next five years regimes that are currently unknown will be demonstrated in centres. These may well require equipment that is now only at the drawing board stage. Not only will jobs be plentiful but there will also be new trends. Physical fitness practitioners will be learning new techniques and about new equipment. The experience may be demanding but it will also surely be exciting and rewarding.

In the hairdressing and the beauty industries, changing fashions and the development of more efficient scientific methods have meant that many techniques have also changed and improved. For example, even during the last five years hair-colouring techniques have changed radically. In the beauty world, airbrushing, a method whereby an airbrush sprays microscopic particles of specially formulated colour that lock on to the skin, is set to revolutionize make-up artists' techniques. The use of electrical and mechanical equipment has both increased and become more sophisticated, requiring a high degree of skill on the part of the beauty therapist, together with an understanding of the scientific principles involved. Specialization is occurring, particularly in the fields of massage and electrolysis; at present, there is a high demand for highly skilled and accurate electrolysists. Trends are constantly changing so it is necessary to update skills at least once every three years.

In all three industries, the future looks good.

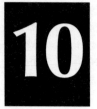

10 Education and training available

Choosing a good training centre

There is a wide range of courses and many different types of training centres in the UK. Check out the following to make sure the training is right for you:

◆ What is the length of the course and is it full- or part-time?
◆ When does the course start?
◆ Is it free or do you have to pay? If you have to pay, are you eligible for a grant?
◆ How many students are on the course and what is the staff/student ratio?
◆ How many students were on the course last year, how many achieved the required level and how many got jobs?
◆ Does the course lead to an approved qualification in your field?
◆ What training route options are available?
◆ If you have to be on a placement, are you given one or do you have to find one yourself?
◆ What level does the course reach?
◆ Does the centre have a quality rating from an external organization?
◆ How much work will you be expected to do every day/week/month?.
◆ Are there exams?

◆ Can you complete the course unit by unit, returning at a convenient time to complete any outstanding units?
◆ Do you have to provide your own equipment and if so how much is this going to cost?
◆ Can you look around the college or training centre and meet the current students and trainers?
◆ How do you enrol? Can you enrol at any time or are there set dates?

Modern Apprenticeship schemes

In the UK, Modern Apprenticeship schemes have been introduced to give capable well-motivated young people access to higher level work-based training. A scheme will take about three years to complete and the final qualifications will include at least an NVQ/SVQ at Level 3 (broadly equivalent to two A levels). They offer work-based training. Training is flexible and adaptable to meet the needs of both employer and employee and the schemes provide an alternative route to higher education. Schemes are available in health and beauty therapy and hairdressing. They are aimed at 16 to 19 year olds who have just left school or college. For further details telephone 0800 100 900, or contact www.dfes.gov.org/modapp/ or your local Skills Council.

National Vocational Qualifications (NVQs) and Scottish Vocational Qualifications (SVQs)

NVQs and SVQs are offered at a large number of centres throughout the UK. They are accessible and open to all ages. The system of awards covers areas of work at specific levels of achievement, and are geared to progression through the different levels. Each contains a series of units, which may be tackled in any order depending on the needs of the individual. Trainees are thus able to progress at their own speed and are assessed when they are ready. NVQs and SVQs are flexible, practical, work-related skills-based qualifications, and achievement is based on demonstrating competence in actually doing a job.

NVQs and SVQs recognize competent performance in a particular job role, and the necessary knowledge and understanding to perform that role effectively. The qualifications are based on standards of competence set by the lead bodies in the industry concerned. They may be awarded at five levels, from Level 1, which covers a range of work activities that are mainly routine and predictable, to Level 5, which covers competence in complex activities often involving significant responsibility for the work of others and for other resources.

Success in a range of units, supported by written and oral work, leads to a Record of Achievement in England and Wales or Record of Education and Training in Scotland. This is assessed in the workplace by assessors, who in turn are backed up by internal and external verifiers. NVQs are accredited by the Qualifications & Curriculum Authority (QCA) in England and Wales and SVQs by the Scottish Qualifications Authority (SQA) in Scotland. SQA is the national body in Scotland responsible for the development, accreditation, assessment and certification of qualifications other than degrees. NVQs/SVQs are available in a wide range of areas and new courses are constantly being developed and accredited. The key and core skill units for Levels 1–4 are as follows:

◆ communication;
◆ application of number;
◆ information technology;
◆ improving own learning and performance;
◆ working with others;
◆ problem solving.

Further information from the Qualifications & Curriculum Authority or the Scottish Qualifications Authority (see page 102).

Training authorities and schemes

England and Wales

In England and Wales, Learning and Skills Councils (formerly Training and Enterprise Councils – TECs) are government-funded bodies with responsibility for ensuring that government training and enterprise initiatives meet local labour market needs. They manage the provision of Modern Apprenticeship schemes. Further information from the Department for Education and Skills.

Scotland

In Scotland, a training programme called Skillseekers Training for Young People has been developed. The programme aims to give young people relevant and transferable skills, a recognized vocational qualification, ideally achieved through the work-based route. The programme is similar in approach to the traditional apprenticeship system. Skillseekers funds training for SQVs for people aged 16–24 and a guarantee of a training place is made to young people aged 16 and 17. Local enterprise companies ensure that training and enterprise initiatives meet local market needs. They manage the Modern Apprenticeships schemes within Skillseekers. Further information from the Scottish Executive, Enterprise and Lifelong Learning Department.

Northern Ireland

In Northern Ireland the Training and Employment Agency was established in 1990 to help jobseekers find employment and to provide people with the relevant skills for work. Jobskills schemes aim to improve the quality of training through NVQ schemes, the main aim being to increase the levels of skill and competence of trainees by obtaining NVQ Levels 1–3. Jobskills schemes are open to 16 and 17 year olds, 18–24 year olds following Modern Apprenticeship schemes in employment, and those up to aged 22 who have a disability. Training is delivered by employers, community organizations, colleges,

67

institutes of further education and training centres. To find out more, go to your local Training and Employment Agency office where a careers officer will provide detailed advice about the types of training available and the names of all the training providers. Further information from Northern Ireland Department of Higher and Further Education, Training and Employment.

Republic of Ireland

The Republic of Ireland's National Traineeship programme, FÁS, is a new system of training tailored to the needs of Irish industry, enterprise and local businesses. It involves alternating periods of training in a FÁS Training Centre and in the employer's workplace. The training content and occupational standards are based on employer consultation and lead to nationally recognized certification. Trainees first develop and learn a range of specific occupational skills in a FÁS training centre. They then move into the employer's workplace where they follow a joint FÁS/Employer agreed schedule of training to develop and enhance their skills to achieve mastery in the workplace and to achieve a formal occupational qualification. Traineeships can last from 6 to 24 months and are open to first-time job seekers and the unemployed. FÁS traineeship courses in hairdressing are currently running in the Athlone Training Centre, Athlone and the Sligo Training Centre, Sligo. Trainee courses in the beauty industry are running in Cork Training Centre, Cork, Tralee Training Centre, Tralee and Galway Training Centre, Galway. Further information from the Republic of Ireland's Foras Áiseanna Saothair (Training and Employment Authority).

Edexcel

Edexcel was created from the union of the University of London Examination Board and the Business & Technology Education Council (BTEC). It provides a wide range of qualifications including GCSEs and A levels, NVQs and BTEC First, National and Higher National Certificates and Diplomas.

Edexcel qualifications are offered in over 6,500 schools and colleges of higher education, and qualifications in hairdressing and beauty therapy are offered.

OCR

Oxford Cambridge and RSA Examinations (OCR) is a new awarding body and provides a full range of vocational and academic qualifications, including NVQs in Sport, Recreation and Allied Occupations.

Training courses for the beauty, fitness and hairdressing industries

Beauty

Aromatherapy

The Aromatherapy Organizations Council (AOC) insists that all accredited training establishments have to train to the requirements as laid down in the core curriculum. The AOC requires a minimum of in-class tuition of 200 hours with additional extensive home study, assignments, supervised practice sessions and case studies. Courses may be full- or part-time. The AOC does not recognize aromatherapy courses taught solely by correspondence. Further information from the AOC.

CIDESCO Diploma in Aromatherapy

This is available only to holders of the International CIDESCO Diploma (see pages 70–72). Candidates are required to have completed a course of at least 90 hours at a registered CIDESCO school covering the aromatherapy training syllabus. On completion of the course, candidates have to produce six case histories and undergo a practical and theoretical exam conducted by the school.

Beauty therapy

The Hairdressing and Beauty Industry Authority (HABIA) in

partnership with City & Guilds offers two levels of NVQs in Beauty Therapy in England, Wales and Northern Ireland. The Scottish Qualifications Authority (SQA) offers three levels of SVQs in Scotland, also in partnership with City & Guilds.

NVQ/SVQ in Beauty Therapy Level 2

This is a nine-unit qualification with one additional unit, which may be taken if desired. The beauty skills areas cover improving facial appearance, using make-up techniques, improving facial skin condition, removing and lightening hair, providing lash and brow treatments and providing and advising on nail care. The additional unit covers ear piercing. Included are three units on supporting health and safety, salon reception duties and maintaining teamwork and a unit on developing positive working relationships with clients.

NVQ/SVQ in Beauty Therapy Level 3

This is a ten-unit qualification, comprising six mandatory units and three from five optional units, with two additional units, which may be taken if desired. The mandatory units cover body massage, providing mechanical and electrical treatments, and improving face and skin conditions using electrical treatments, as well as client service and health, safety and security. There are four optional units covering epilation, aromatherapy, specialist make-up and artificial nail techniques. Additional units cover tanning treatments and dry and wet heat treatments. Further details from HABIA, City & Guilds or SQA.

The following organizations also offer NVQ Levels 2 and 3 in Beauty Therapy: BABTAC, Edexcel, Vocational Training Charitable Trust.

CIDESCO offers a number of courses, including the following:

CIDESCO International Diploma Course

This is widely recognized as the world's best known and most respected beauty qualification. Holders of the CIDESCO Diploma are accepted as having had the finest training, providing skills and knowledge at an international level. The duration of the course is one academic year with a training time of 1,200 hours over three terms at a registered CIDESCO school. On completion of the course students take a number of exams as follows:

Facial exam
◆ cleansing;
◆ skin analysis;
◆ eyelash and eyebrow tinting, eyebrow shaping;
◆ deep cleansing;
◆ electrical equipment;
◆ facial massage;
◆ mask treatment;
◆ make-up, full day make-up;
◆ manicure.

Body exam
◆ body analysis;
◆ electrotherapy;
◆ manual massage;
◆ depilation.

Additional subjects can be chosen from a range of beauty therapy subjects such as:

◆ cellulite treatment;
◆ aromatherapy;
◆ special foot treatment;
◆ anti-stress treatment;
◆ electrical depilation;
◆ fantasy make-up;
◆ lymph drainage.

Written exam
This consists of multiple choice questions from all parts of the CIDESCO theoretical training programme:

- natural science;
- anatomy and physiology
- skin;
- cosmetic science;
- aesthetic treatments;
- business studies.

Practical exam

During the practical exam, great emphasis is placed on professional expertise, hygiene, client care, interaction, and personal presentation.

For further information, contact CIDESCO direct or BABTAC, which is CIDESCO's representative in the UK.

CIBTAC Beauty Therapy and Electrolysis Course

This is seven months full-time or one year part-time. Subjects covered are as follows:

- anatomy and physiology;
- hygiene;
- diet;
- massage;
- electrotherapy;
- epilation;
- heat and light treatment;
- salon management;
- dermatology;
- massage;
- masks;
- make-up;
- theatrical, photographic and television make-up;
- electrolysis;
- depilation;
- slimming treatments;
- skin treatments;
- deportment and grooming;
- eyelash tinting, eyebrow shaping and eyelash extension;
- manicure and pedicure.

For further details, contact BABTAC or CIBTAC.

The International Therapy Examination Council (ITEC) offers a number of courses related to beauty therapy, including the following:

Aestheticienne Diploma

This is an all-inclusive qualification including all aspects of facial work, facial electrical treatments, make-up, manicure/pedicure and waxing. This is a high level course for those considering becoming a beauty specialist. The recommended minimum number of learning hours is 500. There is an exam consisting of case studies, a three-hour theory paper and a practical examination.

Diploma in Physiatrics

This covers all aspects of body treatments, from figure analysis, diet and exercise to body electrical treatments and body massage. It also includes anatomy and physiology. It is a high level course for those wanting to work as a professional in the industry. The recommended minimum number of learning hours is 500. There is an exam consisting of case studies, a three-hour theory paper and a practical exam of one-and-a-half-hours.

Beauty Therapy Diploma

The Beauty Therapy Diploma will be issued to therapists who achieve both the Physiatrics and Aestheticienne Diplomas. This award covers all aspects of beauty treatments: facial treatments, manicure/pedicure, waxing. It is ideal for therapists who wish to work in a salon, health farm, spa, cruise liner or operate their own business. The recommended learning time is a minimum of 50 hours and there is an exam consisting of case studies, a theory paper of three hours and a practical exam of one-and-a-half hours. Further information from ITEC on all of the above three courses.

BTEC National Diploma in Beauty Therapy

This is a full-time two-year course available at colleges of further education. Entry qualifications are usually four GCSEs (grades A–C), including at least one science subject and a subject that demonstrates communication skills (such as English) and another that demonstrates numerical ability (such as maths). Further information from Edexcel.

Body therapy

The Vocational Training Charitable Trust (VTCT) offers a number of courses relating to body therapy, including the following:

VTCT Foundation Course in Anatomy and Physiology

This covers the skeleton and joints, blood and lymphatic systems, muscles and nervous system, endocrine system and breasts, skin and hair. It is a comprehensive qualification, including all that is required in anatomy and physiology for all the NVQs/SVQs.

VTCT Diploma in Anatomy and Physiology

The Diploma course incorporates all the modules of the Foundation Anatomy and Physiology qualification and in addition includes digestive and excretory systems and respiratory and olfactory systems. Further details from the VTCT on the above courses.

CIBTAC provides a Diploma course:

CIBTAC Body Therapist Diploma Course

This course lasts for a minimum of 300 hours and covers the following practical subjects: body massage, electrical treatments, figure analysis, exercises. In addition, the course covers heat treatments, business organization, first aid, salon procedure, ethics and hygiene. There is a three-hour practical exam covering the above subjects and a three-hour written exam. Further details from CIBTAC.

ITAC provides the following course:

ITAC Diploma in Anatomy, Physiology and Massage

This course provides students with a thorough understanding of anatomy and physiology of the body so that they have a complete knowledge of the structure and functions of each area on which they are working. No prerequisite learning is required. Subjects covered are: skeletal system, muscular system, structure of the skin, functions of the skin, skin cancer, vascular system, lymphatic system, neurological system, endocrine system, respiratory system, digestive system, genito-urinary system, reproductive system, body massage, infrared. There are case studies and a three-hour exam paper, together with a 45-minute practical exam. The recommended minimum learning time is 100 hours. Further details from ITAC.

Beautician

CIBTAC offers a number of courses for beauticians, including the following:

CIBTAC Beautician Diploma Course

This course lasts for a minimum of 300 hours and covers the following practical subjects: manicure and pedicure, skin care, face, neck and shoulder massage, eyebrow shaping, eyelash and eyebrow tinting, eyelash extension, face masks, make-up, electrical facial treatments and depilatory waxing. In addition, the course covers business organization, cosmetic science, ethics, first aid, salon procedure and hygiene. There is a three-hour practical exam covering the above subjects and a three-hour written exam. Further details from CIBTAC.

ITEC offers a number of courses, including the following:

ITEC Beauty Specialist Certificate

This qualification equips the holder to work in beauty salons and provide basic facial treatments to clients. No prior knowledge is required. The recommended learning time is 100 hours. Knowledge of the following is required: superficial cleansing, toning, pre-heat treatments, deep cleansing, skin analysis, enhancing the appearance of eyebrows and lashes, eyebrow tweezing, facial massage, masks, structure of the skin, functions of the skin, skin cancer, muscular system, osteology, neurology, angiology (circulatory system), lymphatic system, cosmetic science. There is an exam consisting of case studies and a two-hour theory paper, together with a one-hour practical exam.

ITEC Beauty Specialist Diploma

The Diploma provides a thorough understanding of and skills in facial treatments (omitting electrical treatments), manicure/pedicure and waxing for a beauty specialist requiring a high level qualification in beauty. It is ideal for those seeking employment in salons, health farms and spas. There is no prerequisite knowledge required and the recommended minimum learning time is 350 hours. Subjects covered include the following: toning, pre-heat treatments, deep cleansing, skin analysis, eyebrow tweezing, eyelash perming, facial massage, masks, make-up, application of false eyelashes, waxing, sugaring, bleaching, bust treatments, structure of the skin, histology, muscular system, neurology, structure of the hair and nails, structure of the breast, cosmetic science. There will be an examination of three hours, case studies and a practical exam of two-and-a-half hours. Further details from ITEC on these two courses.

Manicure and pedicure

ITEC Certificate in Manicure and Pedicure

The certificate provides sound background knowledge and practical skills to enable the holder to offer hand and foot treatments. It is also a foundation course for those starting in the beauty industry. No previous knowledge is required. Subjects covered are: manicure and pedicure, osteology, neurology, angiology (circulatory system), lymphatic system, structure of the nail. There are case studies and an exam of two hours, plus three practical exams. The minimum recommended learning time is 50 hours. Further details from ITEC.

Make-up

CIDESCO Diploma in Make-up

Registered CIDESCO colleges of make-up offer courses of at least 950 hours designed to develop existing artistic abilities for anyone wanting to follow a career in professional make-up. Training covers personal fashion, photographic make-up, theatre and film skills, wigwork, hairdressing and period hairstyling, special cosmetic effects and application of prosthesis. Candidates undergo a practical and written exam and are required to write a 2,000-word project during the course. Further details from BABTAC.

ITEC provides the following Diploma:

Diploma in Fashion, Theatre and Media Make-up

This course provides an opportunity to become skilled in make-up for the fashion and entertainment industry. No prior knowledge is required. The subjects covered are: osteology, muscular system, structure of the skin, functions of the skin, skin cancer, lighting, make-up, application of false eyelashes, theatrical make-up. There is a three-hour exam paper and a practical exam of one hour. The recommended minimum learning time is 100 hours. Further details from ITEC.

Film and Television Freelance Training

Film and Television Freelance Training trains people who already have basic make-up and hair qualifications to apply those skills in the specialist field of film and television production. Applicants for training in this area must already have achieved both NVQ/SVQ Level 2 in Hairdressing and Beauty Therapy. Further details from Film and Television Freelance Training.

Skillset

Skillset National Training Organization subsidizes a range of short courses for freelancers and funds new entrant schemes through its Freelance Training Fund and Skills Investment Fund. Up to 60 per cent of the training fees for established freelancers may be paid by Skillset direct to training providers so that they can offer places at a reduced rate.

Skillset and the British Film Institute run a database of over 2,500 short and long courses and there are independent training providers in over 85 locations across the UK. Examples of the courses are as follows: Advanced Fashion Make-up, Body Art, Complete Make-up Artist's Training Programme, Make-up, Film Television and Theatre, Fashion Hair and Make-up, Hair Styles for Make-up Artists, Introduction to Promotional Make-up Techniques, The Guide to Make-Up Artistry, The Guide to Television Make-up Artistry, Face and Body Painting and Ageing for Film and Television. Further details from Skillset.

Beauty consultant

The Vocational Training Charitable Trust (VTCT) offers the following courses:

Customer Service

NVQ and SVQ in Customer Service at Level 2 (Q1051493) and (G62622).
NVQ and SVQ in Customer Service at Level 3 (Q1051500) and (G60L23). Further details of both these courses from the VTCT.

Beauty Consultant Diploma

The International Health and Beauty Council (IHBC), a subsidiary of VTCT, awards a Beauty Consultant Diploma. This is a comprehensive qualification for cosmetic sales persons who need a comprehensive knowledge of make-up and manicure together with the marketing of cosmetics and scents and handling and controlling stock. Further details from VTCT.

ITEC Beauty Consultant Course

ITEC offers a Beauty Consultant course. You have to be aged 18 by the time you sit the examination. Entrance qualifications vary with the individual college, but two GCSEs (A–C) are usually required. Further details from ITEC.

Electrolysis

A reputable electrolysist will become a member of the Institute of Electrolysis. To become a member it is necessary to pass one of the following entry courses: BTEC Higher National Diploma, or National Diploma in Beauty Therapy or NVQ Level 3 or equivalent in epilation. It is then necessary to complete the Institute of Electrolysis Entrance Preparation Three-day Course, and to pass the qualifying entrance exam. All applicants for this exam have to have studied the Institute's syllabus in depth. This comprises in-depth knowledge of the following: anatomy and physiology, including the cardiovascular, lymphatic and endocrine systems; detailed knowledge of the relationship between skin and hair; hygiene and the working environment; diseases and their causes; sterilization and disinfection; client relationship with the electrolysist.

The Institute recommends the following qualifications: NVQ Level 3 in Electrical Epilation, BTEC National Diploma with Epilation, BTEC Higher National Diploma with Epilation.

CIDESCO Diploma in Electrical Epilation

This is available only to holders of the International CIDESCO

Diploma (see above). Candidates are required to have completed a course of at least 200 hours at a registered CIDESCO school. There are practical and theoretical exams.

CIBTAC Electrolysist Diploma Course

This course lasts for a minimum of 300 hours of training if candidates have no previous knowledge of the theory essential for this course. It covers the following subjects: anatomy and physiology, detailed study of the skin and hair, hygiene, basic electricity, care and maintenance of epilation equipment, common skin disorders, salon routine, ethics, business organization, first aid. There is a 20-minute practical exam including oral questions and one written paper of two-and-a-half hours covering the subjects listed above. For further information, contact the Institute of Electrolysis, BABTAC or CIBTAC. The British Association of Electrolysists (BAE) provides advanced training in electrolysis.

Private beauty training schools

There are many private beauty training schools. Some give grounding in the skills and knowledge needed to achieve NVQ/SVQ qualifications. Others allow for career development into specialist beauty skills. Check that the school is approved by QCA or SQA; you might do better to go to your local technical college as some charge a lot of money for not very much training. Contact HABIA for further advice. Three reputable private training schools' courses are listed below:

Champneys International College of Health & Beauty offers courses including the following:

CIDESCO Beauty Therapy Course

This is a full-time course incorporating the full range of the CIDESCO Diploma units (see above), together with CIBTAC and aromatherapy qualifications. The course lasts for 11 months.

CIBTAC Beauty Therapy Course

This is a full-time course incorporating the full range of the CIBTAC course (see above). The course lasts for eight months.

Anatomy, Physiology and Massage

This is a 12-week course leading to a Champneys Diploma.

Anatomy and Physiology

This is a 12-week course leading to a Champneys Diploma.

Champneys Diploma in Nail Treatments (Manicure and Pedicure)

This is a nine-day course. Further information on all these courses from Champneys.

Steiner Beauty Therapy Training offers the following courses:

Beautician Course

This can be taken five days a week full-time, two to three days a week part-time or two evenings a week. Subjects studied are facial skincare treatments, eyebrow shaping, eyelash tinting and application of eyelash extensions, make-up, manicure and pedicure and treatment of superfluous hair. The training time is a minimum of 300 hours. This course of study leads to the Confederation of International Beauty Therapy and Cosmetology Beautician Diploma Examination and School Diploma.

Steiner provides both the CIDESCO syllabus and the CIBTAC syllabus (see pages 70–72) and the following advanced specialized subjects: face and body treatment, aromatherapy with reflexology, Shiatsu acupressure massage, special back treatments, Guinot eye and neck cathiodermie, scalp treatment, remedial cosmetic camouflage make-up, ear-piercing, micro-current dermalift facial. Further information from Steiner.

The Yorkshire College of Beauty Therapy offers a number of courses including the following:

◆ International Aestheticienne/Electrolysis Diploma Course (three terms);
◆ International Aestheticienne Diploma Course (two terms);
◆ Beauty Specialist Diploma Course (one term);
◆ Massage and Body Treatments Course (one term);
◆ Electrolysis Diploma Course (one term);
◆ CIDESCO/ITEC Honours additional hours Diploma Course;
◆ Sports Massage and Injuries Management Course.

Further information from the Yorkshire College of Beauty Therapy.

Fitness

The UK Exercise and Fitness Group, part of SPRITO, recommends that, in order to become fully qualified to teach fitness and exercise disciplines, two stages of personal development are involved. The first stage is the acquisition and development of the basic skills and knowledge in a controlled and safe training environment and the second stage is the application of these skills in a place of employment. The Stage 1 qualifications, provided by OCR, are as follows:

◆ RSA Certificate in Teaching Exercise to Music (note that this course has recently been heavily revised and replaces the RSA Basic Certificate in the Teaching of Exercise to Music);
◆ RSA Certificate in Teaching Aqua;
◆ RSA Certificate in Teaching Gym;
◆ RSA Certificate in Teaching Circuits;
◆ RSA Certificate in Teaching Step.

The following NVQs, awarded by OCR, are relevant for a qualification in fitness:

Sport, Recreation and Allied Occupations Level 1

This is for new entrants to the sport and recreation sector who work in a range of facilities and environments. There are six mandatory units:

◆ prepare activities within a session;
◆ lead activities within a session;
◆ help to provide activities;
◆ help to maintain facility areas;
◆ help to maintain good working relationships;
◆ deal with accidents and emergencies.

Sport, Recreation and Allied Occupations: Coaching, Teaching and Instructing Level 2

This is for people undertaking some basic training in coaching, teaching and instructing and who now wish to develop themselves as professional coaches. The qualification is assessed and certificated in the context of a specific sporting activity as follows: music, step, circuits, gymnasium, aqua and fitness. The basic course contents for an NVQ/SVQ Level 2 for fitness instruction are as follows:

◆ study of anatomy and physiology and their relevance to the discipline taught;
◆ how to teach safe exercises with good technique;
◆ sound teaching methods;
◆ principles of training and safe programme design;
◆ lesson planning;
◆ planning progressive programmes;
◆ health and safety;
◆ customer care, promoting physical activity;
◆ safe teaching methods.

Sport, Recreation and Allied Occupations: Operational Services Level 2

This is for those who work in sport and leisure facilities as part of a team responsible for the delivery of a range of customer

services (including leading fitness sessions) and/or the maintenance of equipment and plant. There are five mandatory units:

- deal with accidents and emergencies;
- develop and maintain positive working relationships with customers;
- make information and advice available to customers;
- support the work of a team;
- contribute to maintaining a safe and secure environment.

There are four optional units from the following:

- maintain the safety of swimming pool users;
- operate plant to maintain levels of heating and ventilation;
- operate plant to maintain the quality of pool water;
- operate plant to provide and maintain an ice surface;
- maintain sport and recreation equipment and facilities;
- provide equipment for activities;
- solve problems for customers;
- receive customers and visitors;
- contribute to developing own and organizational practice;
- clean and tidy sport and recreation areas;
- deal with substances hazardous to health;
- prepare for coaching sessions;
- conduct coaching sessions;
- promote the adoption and maintenance of regular physical activity.

Sport, Recreation and Allied Occupations: Operations and Development Level 3

This is for those who work in sport and leisure facilities or in
the delivery of sports development services who have consider-
able responsibility, which may include supervisory management. There are six mandatory units:

- promote a culture of health and safety;
- managing yourself;
- create effective working relationships;

◆ support the efficient use of resources;
◆ plan and organize services and operations to meet expectations and requirements;
◆ solve problems on behalf of customers.

There are four optional units from the following:

◆ organize travel for participants and equipment;
◆ support the protection of children from abuse;
◆ supervise residential experiences;
◆ enable people with disabilities to take part in activities;
◆ contribute to the development of teams and individuals;
◆ respond to poor performance in your team;
◆ contribute to the selection of personnel for activities;
◆ manage information for action;
◆ contribute to marketing, developing and promoting services;
◆ maximize product sales;
◆ help customers to choose between products;
◆ maintain reliable customer service;
◆ maintain sport and recreation equipment and facilities;
◆ operate plant to maintain levels of heating and ventilation;
◆ operate plant to maintain the quality of pool water;
◆ operate plant to provide and maintain an ice surface.

Development Training, Level 3

This is aimed at those involved in designing and delivering development training in the outdoors, often working with adults and young people to meet development objectives of client organizations. There are five mandatory units:

◆ contribute to improving personal and organizational performance;
◆ promote a culture of health and safety;
◆ promote the conservation of the environment;
◆ organize people and resources for outdoor programmes;
◆ establish and maintain effective working relationships.

There are four optional units from the following:

◆ support the efficient use of resources;
◆ design outdoor education programmes;
◆ deliver education in the outdoors;
◆ promote the transfer of learning from outdoor experiences;
◆ design outdoor development training programmes;
◆ deliver development training in the outdoors;
◆ deliver recreation in the outdoors;
◆ plan outdoor recreation programmes;
◆ lead the work of teams and individuals to achieve their objectives;
◆ organize travel for participants and equipment;
◆ support the protection of children from abuse;
◆ supervise residential experiences;
◆ enable people with disabilities to take part in activities;
◆ facilitate adventurous experiences;
◆ facilitate participant investigation and understanding of the environment.

Further information from SPRITO or OCR.

BTEC HNC/D Leisure Management, Sport and Recreation and Outdoor Activities

These courses are for the sixth-form leaver and anyone wanting a career change. You must be aged 18 or over and have at least one A level or equivalent. Each course lasts for two years in a continuous process undertaken via a number of assignments. The following units are included in the course: business systems in leisure, management of people in leisure, managing finance in leisure, marketing and sales for the leisure industry, sports promotion, customer care and service quality, outdoor activities, lifestyle and well-being, health promotion and fitness, principles of sports coaching, special populations in health and fitness, technology in sport and leisure, water-based activities, countryside and the environment, small business enterprise. Further information from Edexcel.

ITEC provides a number of courses related to fitness, including the following:

ITEC Diploma in Fitness and Sports Therapy

This covers a wide range of fitness and sports therapy subjects that show the holder has extensive knowledge and skill as a sports therapist and fitness instructor. The award requires the graduate to have passed at least six subjects in anatomy and physiology, sports massage, sports therapy equipment, aerobics teaching, diet and nutrition and personal training. To undertake the course you must have a current first-aid certificate. The recommended minimum number of learning hours is 450. There are case studies, a three-hour exam paper and a 45-minute practical exam.

ITEC Diploma in Gym Instruction

Before undertaking this course, students must hold the ITEC Diploma in Anatomy, Physiology and Massage (see page 92). Subjects covered are anatomy and physiology, fitness testing and screening and training methods. There are case studies and a three-hour exam and one-hour practical exam. The recommended minimum learning time is three hours.

ITEC Diploma in Aerobics Teaching

Before undertaking this course, students must hold the ITEC Diploma in Anatomy, Physiology and Massage (see page 92). This course provides a full understanding of the muscular system and the cardiovascular system, so that students are able to advise clients on the importance of warm-up, cool-down, stretching and prevention of injuries. The course teaches choreography and exercise to music. Subjects covered are nutrition and diet, fitness testing and screening and aerobics. There are case studies and a three-hour exam as well as a 30-minute practical exam. The recommended minimum number of learning hours is 50.

ITEC Personal Trainer's Diploma

Before taking this course, students must hold the ITEC Diploma in Aerobics Teaching, the ITEC Gym Instructors' Certificate and the ITEC Diploma in Diet and Nutrition, as well as a current first-aid certificate. Subjects covered are: nutrition, exercise psychology, programme design, communication skills, clients' health problems, environment, teaching techniques and safety. There are case studies and a three-hour exam paper. The recommended minimum number of learning hours is 50. Further details on all four courses from ITEC.

The IIHHT, part of the VTCT, provides a number of qualifications in massage, including a Body Massage Diploma, a Remedial Massage Diploma and a Sports Massage Certificate. There are also four courses in Health and Fitness Studies.

Diploma in Health and Fitness Studies

This course incorporates a core of nine modules covering employment, anatomy and physiology and nutrition as well as exercise to music, circuit training, basic fitness testing and gymnasium-based exercise. Further information from VTCT.

The Institute of Sport and Recreation Management (ISRM) provide a number of courses including the following:

Supervisory Management Certificate

This course is for sport and recreation facility supervisors. It provides the underpinning knowledge leading to the NVQ/SVQ Level 3 in Sport and Recreation Supervision. Each module is a separate course and a certificate is awarded on successful completion. The following four modules must be successfully completed:

- sports facility operations;
- supervision and leadership;
- finance and administration;
- practice and employment.

Sport and Recreation Management Certificate

This is a nationally recognized qualification for the management of sports halls, leisure centres and swimming pools. The qualification consists of four modules:

◆ design and technical operations;
◆ activity operations and general law;
◆ administration and management;
◆ sport and recreation management.

Each module is assessed by a three-hour written paper. Further details from ISRM.

FitPro provides a number of courses for fitness instructors and personal trainers, including the following:

AIM (Advanced Instructor Modules)

The modules are designed for instructors already in possession of a health or exercise qualification who are looking to diversify their skills and enhance their knowledge. At least two years' working experience within the aerobics/fitness industry is required, along with a sound base of knowledge relevant to the module. Each module is presented by qualified educators and provides comprehensive workbooks and a Certificate of Attendance.

Attendees will have the opportunity to sit a theoretical exam at the end of the module that will assess underpinning knowledge. Results and a certificate of achievement will be forwarded to the participants following successful completion of the exam.

Case studies are also available, giving candidates the opportunity to apply the practical knowledge they have learnt throughout the module in a 'real life' scenario. Successful completion of each assessment will contribute towards the provision of evidence for specific elements of the NVQ/SVQ Level 3. Further details from FitPro.

The YMCA Fitness Industry Training runs a number of exercise instructor training courses including the following:

Professional Studio Instructor Award

◆ step 1 – exercise and fitness knowledge module;
◆ step 2 – exercise to music (aerobics);
◆ step 3 – compulsory module (to choose one of four);
◆ studio resistance training;
◆ group indoor cycling;
◆ step choreography;
◆ aqua exercise.

To receive the Professional Studio Instructor Award Certificate you will also need a current Emergency Medical Planning Certificate.

Professional Gym Instructor Award

◆ step 1 – exercise and fitness knowledge module;
◆ step 2 – gym training;
◆ step 3 – compulsory module (to choose one of three);
◆ studio resistance training;
◆ group indoor cycling;
◆ circuit training.

To receive the Professional Gym Instructor Award Certificate you will also need a current Emergency Medical Planning Certificate. Further information from the YMCA Fitness Industry Training.

The Medau Movement runs a teacher training course. Spread over five terms the integrated syllabus includes:

◆ movement training, including personal performance, breathing and relaxation;
◆ underpinning knowledge, including anatomy, physiology, first aid and health and safety;
◆ teaching skills;
◆ teaching resources, including movement, percussion and recorded music.

Further information from the Medau Movement.

Fitness therapies

The Alexander Technique

The Society of Teachers of the Alexander Technique (STAT) currently (2001) offers 12 courses in the UK with a three-year training course. All accredited courses must offer at least 1,600 hours of tuition over a period of three years. There are three terms and classes are held on average for four hours including breaks, four or five days a week. Students have to undertake additional study in their own time and need to be able to organize their routine of work and practice without undue stress and fatigue. It is essential for students to know how to employ the technique personally before they can learn to teach it to others.

In class, the work is mainly of a practical nature and instruction is usually given individually or in small groups – the student–teacher ratio is never more than five to one. Time is provided for lectures or discussions on relevant basic anatomy and physiology and a wide course of reading is recommended according to the special needs and interests of the individual. Further information from STAT.

Feldenkrais

The Feldenkrais International Training Centre Ltd offers an accredited training course to become a Feldenkrais practitioner/teacher, on a part-time programme spread over three to four years. This is divided into full-time segments each year, usually about 40 days per year. There are no specific requirements or qualifications required to be eligible for a training programme, but you are expected to have had personal experience of the methods and to have taken lessons before deciding to commit yourself to the training.

When you have completed the training programme you will be a graduate of a professional training programme accredited by the European Training Accreditation Board of the

International Feldenkrais Federation. Your diploma will qualify you for membership of the national professional guilds and associations of Feldenkrais teachers worldwide. You will be qualified to teach the Feldenkrais Method to the public and to give individual lessons. Further information from the Feldenkrais International Training Centre.

Massage

ITEC offers a number of courses in massage including the following:

Diploma in Anatomy, Physiology and Massage

This course lasts about 100 hours. It provides students with a thorough understanding of anatomy and physiology of the body so that they have a complete knowledge of the structure and functions of each area on which they are working. Holistic massage is included. There is an exam at the end of the course. No prerequisite learning is required.

Diploma in Sports Massage

This course lasts for about 35 hours. It enables the therapist to understand the effects and benefits of massage to assist in dealing with injury and training requirements. The qualification is useful for those who want to work in leisure centres and with sports clubs and competitive athletes and teams. The prerequisites for the course are the ITEC Diploma in Anatomy, Physiology and Massage or the ITEC Diploma in Physiatrics (see page 73). Further information from ITEC.

Pilates

The training course for Pilates teachers normally consists of between one and three years, depending on whether the course is taken part- or full-time. A typical course comprises a minimum of one year with a minimum of 300 hours of theoretical work on the syllabus, followed by six months' apprenticeship with a minimum of 20 hours per week of supervised teaching practice. If you want to be a Pilates teacher you should have a background in exercise and/or movement and should have completed 25–30 Pilates studio sessions before you start your training.

There are 36 Pilates studios in the UK but not all of these offer training. The following, however, do offer training: Backlund Pilates has two intakes per year and training takes place in the studio on Tuesdays and Wednesdays between 10 am and 4 pm. The Pilates and Yoga Movement Studio takes on three full-time students per year. Part-time courses over 1,200 hours are also offered followed by a six-month apprenticeship of 20 hours per week. Belsize Studio has two intakes per year and South-east Pilates Exercise Centre is starting teacher training courses for groups of approximately 10 people at a time from January 2002. Applications for the first course open in September 2001. Further information from the above-mentioned centres and from the Pilates Foundation.

T'ai Chi Chuan

At present (2001), there are no recognized training centres as such for this martial art. Potential practitioners join a centre where they learn their craft hands-on, guided by experienced practitioners. Four recommended institutions are Practical Tai Chi Chuan, T'ai Chi UK, Herts Long Fei Taijiquan Association and the Tai Chi Union.

Yoga

The British School of Yoga (BSY) offers a number of courses nationwide. Each course consists of a number of lessons that are both self-contained yet part of the whole course. A test paper is set at the end of each lesson that is marked and corrected by your tutor. This way, you can be sure that you have mastered each aspect of your course before moving on to the next. For further information, write to the BSY asking for details and enclosing an sae.

The British Wheel of Yoga offers a diploma course available in over 50 venues throughout England, Scotland and Wales. The course is part-time, comprising of around 150 hours of tuition, and lasts for about two-and-a-half years. It leads to the British Wheel of Yoga Teacher's Diploma. The syllabus covers the practice and teaching of Hatha yoga techniques, relaxation and meditation, and basic anatomy and physiology. Theoretical study includes four set books: The *Bhagavad Gita*, the *Upanishads*, the *Yoga Sutras of Pantanjali* and the *Hathayoga Pradipika*. The syllabus also covers the area of professional studies, that is, learning about how to teach and plan courses and lessons. Contact the British Wheel of Yoga for further details.

The Iyengar Yoga Institute offers a two-year part-time course consisting of a minimum of 120 hours of classes. At the end of the first year having completed 60 hours' training, you will sit the Part 1 assessment of the Introductory certificate and the Part 2 at the end of the second year and completion of 120 hours. Before you are accepted for enrolment in an Iyengar Yoga teacher-training class you must have regularly attended the classes of a fully recognized Iyengar Yoga teacher who must provide a written recommendation that will confirm you have attended classes regularly for a minimum of four years (five from 2003). Contact the Iyengar Yoga Institute for further details.

Hairdressing

The Hairdressing and Beauty Industry Authority (HABIA), in partnership with City & Guilds, offers three levels of National Vocational Qualifications (NVQs) in Hairdressing in England, Wales and Northern Ireland (Hairdressing NVQ Scheme Number 3017). The Scottish Qualifications Authority (SQA) offers three levels of Scottish Vocational Qualifications (SVQs) in Scotland, also in partnership with City & Guilds (Hairdressing SVQ Scheme Number 3018). These are the main qualifications in hairdressing.

Level 1

This is an introduction to the hairdressing industry and is suitable for school work experience and junior staff induction. It is based on assisting technical staff. When you work towards

Level 1 standards, you will be covering the basic skills required in every salon by all hairdressers, under the supervision of more experienced staff in the salon. You will help to run the salon by performing such tasks as:

◆ shampoo, condition and dry hair;
◆ assist with perming, relaxing and colouring hair;
◆ help with attending to clients and enquiries;
◆ help to make sure the health and safety regulations in the salon are adhered to.

Level 2

This is the standard qualification for stylists and barbers and covers the basic skills and knowledge required to become a competent hairdresser. It is the minimum required for becoming a State Registered Hairdresser (see page 12). The skills cover the range of hairdressing services offered by a salon such as:

◆ shampooing and conditioning hair and scalp;
◆ blow-drying and cutting;
◆ perming, relaxing and neutralizing;
◆ setting and dressing;
◆ colouring;
◆ use of resources;
◆ barbering;
◆ health and safety;
◆ reception duties;
◆ working relationships;
◆ client care.

Level 3

This is an advanced qualification, equivalent to an A level. It is aimed at barbers, senior stylists and technicians, as well as those wishing to gain supervisory skills and become involved in staff training, who want to expand and develop their skills and responsibilities. It covers the following subjects:

- cutting, including fashion cutting, perming and colouring;
- training and supervisory skills;
- African Caribbean hairdressing;
- improving systems and procedures.

There is another level, Level 4 NVQ in Hairdressing, currently offered only by HABIA, which is aimed at salon managers. It does not expand on technical hairdressing skills. This is based on nationally recognized standards developed by the Management and Enterprise National Training Organizations. It includes the following:

- business planning;
- marketing;
- personnel and financial planning for salons.

The following organizations also award NVQs or SVQs in Hairdressing: Edexcel, VTCT. CIBTAC offers the following courses:

Foundation Modern Apprenticeship in Hairdressing

Open to 16–18-year-old school leavers. People aged over 18 may also be eligible as long as they can complete by their 25th birthday. The target qualification is NVQ/SVQ Level 2 and the scheme is likely to last two-and-a-half years. There is funding assistance available.

Advanced Modern Apprenticeships in Hairdressing

Open to 16–18-year-old school leavers. People aged over 18 may also be eligible as long as they can complete by their 25th birthday. The target qualification is NVQ/SVQ Level 3 and the scheme is likely to last three-and-a-half years. There is funding assistance available.

Assistant Beautician Certificate Course

This course is designed for the benefit of the student attending a full-time hairdressing course in a technical college. It covers instruction in such beauty treatments as can be efficiently and safely carried out in a hairdressing salon and provides an additional qualification to a professional hairdresser. Candidates must have practical and theoretical knowledge of the following: manicuring and pedicuring, disorders of the nails, skin care, make-up, eyebrow shaping, eyelash and eyebrow tinting and depilatory waxing. The course is designed to last for a minimum of 125 hours and it mostly consists of practical work. There is a two-and-a-half-hour practical exam and a two-hour written exam. Further information from CIBTAC.

Other hairdressing training organizations

Hairdressing Trainers Organization

There are five training centres in Essex. The student, known as a Modern Apprentice, is employed by a hairdressing organization while working towards the NVQ Levels 2 and 3, in addition to learning personal skills. There is a thorough selection process to identify high-calibre motivated young people. Full training and support are given to enhance their knowledge and awareness of the business. The training is structured over a three-and-a-half-year period to enable the young person to develop. You will be given a training schedule at the start of the programme and there is a mixture of off-the-job training sessions and on-the-job monitoring visits.

Skillset

This is the national training organization for broadcast, film, video and interactive media. It subsidizes a range of short courses for freelances and funds new entrance schemes through its Freelance Training Fund and Skills Investment Fund. Up to 60 per cent of the training fees for established freelances can be paid by Skillset direct to training providers so that they can offer places to freelancers at a reduced rate. Skillset and the British

Film Institute have developed and run a database of over 2,500 long and short courses in further and higher education within industry, and with independent training providers in over 85 locations throughout the UK. Courses in hairdressing are as follows:

◆ Complete Make-Up Artist's Training Programme;
◆ Period Wigs and Hair;
◆ Fashion Hair and Make-up;
◆ Fashion Hair Styling;
◆ Hair for Stage, Film and Television;
◆ Hair Styles for Make-up Artists;
◆ Make-up and Hairdressing – Total Look Fashion;
◆ NVQ Level 3: Long Hair, Wig and Hair Piece Design – Attachment
◆ Total Look for Media to Television;
◆ Film, Television and Fashion Make-up and Hair;
◆ Professional Make-up Skills including Hair and Face-Painting.

Steiner Training Ltd

Steiner Training is an interview and recruitment organization for Steiner Transocean Ltd. They employ only fully qualified people for the hairdressing salons. New employees are then trained up to Steiner's specific requirements.

Trichology

Training

To become a recognized trichologist you should become a member of the Institute of Trichologists. To become a member you have to take the Institute's three-year Trichology course. This is academic and scientific in nature and requires great commitment and motivation, particularly because it is not a full-time course. Entry requirements are passes in a minimum of four GCSEs grade C or above, or Grade 1 in the General Scottish Certificate of Secondary Education. Subjects must include English language, maths and a science. Passes in two subjects at A level are also necessary or successful completion of the Institute of Trichologists' Foundation Course.

Foundation Course

This is a six-month distance learning programme comprising theoretical and academic study only; there is no practical element to the course. Studies include: anatomy and physiology, inorganic chemistry, scalp and hair and the nature and scope of trichology. Examinations are held twice-yearly and comprise one three-hour written paper, based on material contained within the course modules.

Three-Year Course in Trichology

The distance learning course is in three parts, known as levels, each normally taking one year to complete. It includes study of the following topics: anatomy and physiology (human biology), basic microbiology, genetics, anatomy and physiology of the scalp and hair, processing of hair, hygiene, inorganic chemistry, trichological procedures, massage, nutrition, organic chemistry, trichological preparations, micro-diagnostic techniques, basic physics, electrotherapy, statistics, hair disorders, hair loss, hirsutism, scalp disorders, and organization and operation of a trichological practice. Examinations comprise one three-hour written paper for Level 1; two three-hour papers for Level 2 and two three-hour papers, a practical examination and an oral examination for Level 3.

The course material comprises modules published by the Institute and sent to you to keep. You do not need to buy any other books or printed materials. You are also assigned a personal tutor who will monitor your progress and mark your submitted assignments. There are various assignments to complete and return to your tutor for marking and assessment. For example in the first year at Level 1 you will have to complete 16 assignments and submit these for marking and assessment. You will be expected to attend two one-day seminars during each year of the course and during the later stages of the course, students are invited to attend for clinical training and observation at an approved clinic of a practising member of the Institute. Further information from the Institute of Trichologists.

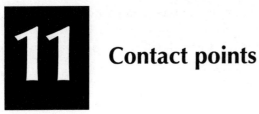

Contact points

General

City & Guilds of London Institute – Head Office
1 Giltspur Street, London EC1A 9DD; Tel: (020) 7294 2468,
Fax: (020) 7294 2412, www.city-and-guilds.co.uk

City & Guilds – regional office
Eastern
Tel: (01223) 426422

East Midlands
Tel:(01773) 842900

London and South East
Tel: (020) 7294 2820

North East and Cumbria
Tel: (0191) 402 5100

North West
Tel: (01925) 820006

Northern Ireland and Republic of Ireland
Tel: (022890) 325689

Scotland
Tel: (0131) 226 1556

South West
Tel: (01823) 722200

Southern England
Tel: (020) 7294 2724

Wales
Tel: (02920) 265190

West Midlands
Tel: (0121) 359 6667

Department for Education and Skills (DfES), Sanctuary Buildings, Great Smith Street, London SW1P 3BT; Tel: (0870) 000 2288, Fax: (0192) 879 4248, Email: info@dfes.gsi.gov.uk, www.dfes.gov.uk

Edexcel, Stewart House, 32 Russell Square, London WC1B 5DN; Tel: (0870) 240 9800, Fax: (020) 7758 6960, Email: enquiries@edexcel.org.uk, www.edexcel.org.uk

International Therapy Examination Council (ITEC), 10–11 Heathfield Terrace, Chiswick, London W4 4JE; Tel: (020) 8994 4141, Fax: (020) 8994 7880, Email: info@itecworld.co.uk, www.itecworld.co.uk

Northern Ireland Department of Higher and Further Education, Training and Employment, Adelaide House, Adelaide Street, Belfast BT2 8FD; Tel: (028) 9025 7777, Fax: (028) 9025 7778, Email: info.tea@nics.gov.uk, www.nics.gov.uk

Oxford Cambridge and RSA Examinations (OCR), Customer Information Bureau, OCR Coventry Office, Westwood Way, Coventry CV4 8JQ; Tel: (02476) 470033, Fax: (02476) 468080, Email: cib@ocr.org.uk

Qualifications & Curriculum Authority (QCA), 83 Piccadilly, London W1J 8QA; Tel: (020) 7509 5555, www.qca.org.uk

Republic of Ireland Foras Áiseanna Saothair, Training and Employment Authority, PO Box 456, 27–33 Upper Baggot Street, Dublin 4; Tel: (1) 6070 500, Fax: (1) 6070 600, Email: info@fas.ie, www.fas.ie

Scottish Executive, Enterprise and Lifelong Learning Department, Meridian Court, Glasgow G2 6AT; Tel: (0141) 248 4774, Fax: (0141) 242 5665, Email: ceu@scotland.gov.uk, www.scotland.gov.uk

Scottish Qualifications Authority (SQA), Hanover House, 24 Douglas Street, Glasgow G2 7NQ; Tel: (0141) 242 2214, Fax: (0141) 242 2244, Email: helpdesk@sqa.org.uk, www.sqa.org.uk

Vocational Training Charitable Trust (VTVC), Head Office, 3rd Floor, Eastleigh House, Upper Market Street, Eastleigh, Hampshire SO50 9FD; Tel: (02380) 684500, Fax: (02380) 651493, www.vtct.org.uk

Beauty

British Association of Beauty Therapy and Cosmetology, BABTAC House, 70 Eastgate Street, Gloucester GL1 1QN; Tel: (01452) 421114, Fax: (01452) 421110, www.babtac.com

British Association of Massage Practitioners, 78 Meadow Street, Preston, Lancashire PR1 1TS; Tel: (01772) 881063, Fax: (01772) 881063, Email: Jolanta@Jolanta.co.uk, www.jolanta.co.uk

BBC Corporation Recruitment Services, PO Box 7000, London W12 7ZY; Tel: (020) 7580 4468

Champneys International College of Health & Beauty, Wigginton, Tring, Hertfordshire HP23 6HY; Tel: (01442) 291333, Fax: (01442) 291334, Email: college@champneys. co.uk, www.champneys.com

Comité International d'Esthetique et de Cosmetologie, Secretariat Witikonerstrasse 365 CH-8053, Zurich, Switzerland; Tel: (01) 380 0075, Fax: (01) 380 0105, Cidsec@access.ch, www.cidesco.com

Confederation of International Beauty Therapy and Cosmetology (CIBTAC), BABTAC House, 70 Eastgate Street, Gloucester GL1 1QN; Tel: (01452) 421114, Fax: (01452) 421110, www.cibtec.com

Film and Television Freelance Training, 4th Floor, Warwick House, 9 Warwick Street, London W1B 5LY; Tel: (020) 7734 5141, www.ft2.org.uk

Guild of Professional Beauty Therapists, Guild House, PO Box 310, Derby DE23 9BR; Tel: (0870) 000 4242, Fax: (0870) 000 4247, www.beautyserve.com

Hairdressing and Beauty Industry Authority (HABIA), Fraser House, Nether Hall Road, Doncaster DN1 2PH; Tel: (01302) 380000, Fax: (01302) 380028, Email: enquiries@habia.org.uk, www.habia.org.uk

Hairdressing & Beauty Suppliers Organization (HBSA), 2nd Floor, Bedford Chambers, The Piazza, Covent Garden, London WC2E 8HA; Tel: (020) 7836 4008, Fax: (020) 7379 1514, www.hbsa.uk.com

International Federation of Health and Beauty Therapists, 3rd Floor, Eastleigh House, Upper Market Street, Eastleigh, Hampshire SO50 9FD; Tel: (023) 8048 8900, Fax: (023) 8048 8970, www.fht.org.uk

International Health and Beauty Council, Unit 11, Brickfield Trading Estate, Brickfield Lane, Chandlers Ford, Hampshire SO53 4DR; Tel: (023) 8027 1733, Fax: (023) 8027 0566

International Nail Association, Guild House, PO Box 310, Derby DE23 9BR; Tel: (0870) 000 4242

London College of Fashion, 20 John Prince's Street, London W1M OBJ;Tel: (020) 7514 7400

Skillset National Training Organization, 2nd Floor, 103 Dean Street, London W1V 5RA; Tel: (020) 7534 5300; Tel: (020) 7534 5333, Email: info@skillset.org, www.skillset.org

Steiner Beauty Therapy Training, 193 Wardour Street, London W1V 3FA;Tel: (020) 7434 4534, Fax: (020) 7434 4544

Steiner Training Ltd, 92 Uxbridge Road, Harrow Weald, Middlesex HA3 6BZ;Tel: (020) 8909 5016

Vocational Training Charitable Trust, Unit 11 Brickfield Trading Estate, Brickfield Lane, Chandlers Ford, Hampshire SO53 4DR;Tel: (023) 8027 1733, Fax: (023) 8027 0566

Yorkshire College of Beauty Therapy, Dragons Health Club, Haworth Lane, Yeadon, Leeds LS19 7EN; Tel: (0113) 250 9507, Fax: (0113) 250 8781, Email: info@ycob.co.uk, www.ycob.co.uk

Aromatherapy

Aromatherapy Organizations Council, PO Box 19834, London SE25 6WF; Tel: (020) 8251 7912, Fax: (020) 8251 7942, www.aoc.uk.net

Electrolysis

British Association of Electrolysists (BAE), 40 Park Field Road, Ickenham, Middlesex UB10 8LW;Tel: (0870) 1280477, Email: sec@baeltd.fsbusiness.co.uk

The Institute of Electrolysis Ltd, PO Box 5187, Milton Keynes MK4 2ZF; Tel: (01908) 521511, Email: institute@electrolysis. co.uk, www.electrolysis.co.uk

Hydrotherapy

Association and Register of Colon Hydrotherapists, 16 Drummond Ride, Tring, Hertfordshire HP23 5DE; Tel: (01442) 825 632, Fax: (01442) 827 687, www.colonic-association.com

Fitness

British Association for Sport and Exercise Sciences (BASES), 114 Cardigan Road, Headingley, Leeds LS6 3BJ; Tel: (0113) 289 1020, Fax: (0113) 231 9606, www.bases.co.uk

Central Council of Physical Recreation (CCPR), Francis House, Francis Street, London SW1P 1DE; Tel: (020) 7854 8500, Fax: (020) 7854 8501, Email: admin@ccpr.org.uk, www.ccpr.org.uk

Federation of Holistic Therapies, 3rd Floor, Eastleigh House, Upper Market Street, Eastleigh, Hampshire SO50 9FD; Tel: (023) 8048 8900, Fax: (023) 8048 8970, Email: info@fht.org.uk, www.fht.org.uk

Fitness Industry Association, 5–11 Lavington Street, London SE1 0NZ; Tel: (020) 7620 0700, www.fia.org.uk

Fitness League, 52 London Street, Chertsey, Surrey KT16 8AJ; Tel: (01932) 564 567, Fax: (01932) 567 566, www.thefitnessleague.com

Fitness Northern Ireland, 147 Holywood Road, Belfast BT4 3BE; Tel: (028) 906 51103

Fitness Professionals (FitPro), 107–113 London Road, London E13 ODA; Tel: (0990) 133 0685, Fax: (020) 8586 0685, Email: admin@fitpro.com, www.fitpro.com

Fitness Recruitment Ltd, PO Box 1881, Stanford-le-Hope, Essex SS17 7FE; Tel: (01375) 679477, Fax: (01375) 679488, www.fitnessrecruitment.net

Fitness Scotland, Caledonia House, South Gyle, Edinburgh EH12 9DQ; Tel: (0131) 317 7243, Fax: (0131) 317 1998, Email: fitscot@talk21.com, www.fitness-scotland.com

Fitness Wales, Nwyfiant Cymru, 240 Whitchurch Road, Cardiff CF41 3ND; Tel: (029) 205 20130, Fax: (029) 206 23152, Email: enquiries@fitnesswales.co.uk, www.fitnesswales.co.uk

International Association of Margaret Morris Movement Ltd, PO Box 1525, Helensburgh, Dunbartonshire G84 0AF, Email: info@margaretmorrismovement.com, www.margaretmorrismovement.com

International Council of Health, Fitness and Sports Therapists, 3rd Floor, Eastleigh House, Upper Market Street, Eastleigh, Hampshire SO50 9FD; Tel: (023) 8048 8900, Fax: (023) 8048 8900, www.fht.org.uk

International Institute of Health & Holistic Therapies (IIHHT), Unit 11, Brickfield Trading Estate, Brickfield Lane, Chandlers Ford, Hampshire SO53 4DR; Tel: (023) 8027 1733, Fax: (023) 8027 0566

Institute of Sport and Recreation Management, Giffard House, 36–38 Sherrard Street, Melton Mowbray, Leicestershire LE13 1XJ; Tel: (01664) 565531, Email: ralphriley@isrm.co.uk, www.isrm.co.uk

Keep Fit Association (KFA); Tel: (020) 8692 9566; or Tel: (020) 8671 8464

Medau Movement, 8b Robson House, East Street, Epsom, Surrey KT17 1HH; Tel: (01372) 729056, Fax: (01372) 729056, Email: medau@nascr.net, www.medau.org.uk

National Training Organization for Sport, Recreation and Allied Occupations (SPRITO), 24 Stephenson Way, London NW1 2HD; Tel: (020) 7388 7755, www.sprito.org.uk

Physical Education Association of the UK, Ling House, Building 25, London Road, Reading RG1 5AQ; Tel: (0118) 931 6240, www.pea.uk.com

Sports Coach UK, 114 Cardigan Road, Headingley, Leeds LS6 3BJ; Tel: (0113) 274 4802, Fax: (0113) 275 5019, Email: fhs@sportscoachuk.org, www.sportscoachuk.org

Sport England, 16 Upper Woburn Place, London WC1H 0QP; Tel: (020) 7273 1500, Fax: (020) 7273 1868, Email: info@english.sports.gov.uk, www.english.sports.gov.uk

Sportscotland, Caledonia House, South Gyle, Edinburgh EH12 9DQ; Tel: (0131) 317 7200, Fax: (0131) 317 7202, www.ssc.org.uk

Sports Council for Northern Ireland, House of Sport, Upper Malone Road, Belfast BT9 5LA; Tel: (028) 9038 1222, www.sportni.org.uk

Sports Council for Wales, Welsh Institute of Sport, Sophia Gardens, Cardiff CF1 9SW; Tel: (029) 2030 0500, Fax: (029) 2030 0600, www.sports.wales.co.uk

Steiner Transocean, The Lodge, 92 Uxbridge Road, Harrow Weald, Middlesex HA3 6BZ; Tel: (020) 8909 5016, www.steinerleisure.com

Vocational Training Charitable Trust, Unit 11, Brickfield Trading Estate, Chandlers Ford, Hampshire SO53 4DR; Tel: (023) 8027 1733, Fax: (023) 8027 0566

YMCA Fitness Industry Training, 111 Great Russell Street, London WC1B 3NP; Tel: (020) 7343 1850, Fax: (020) 7436 1278, www.central@centralymcafit.org.uk

YMCA Fitness Industry Training – Scotland, 9 Lounsdale Avenue, The Oval, Paisley PA2 9LT; Tel: (0141) 889 6208

Fitness Therapies

Alexander Technique

Alexander Technique, Society of Teachers of the Alexander Technique, 129 Camden Mews, London NW1 9AH; Tel: (020) 7284 3338, Fax: (020) 7482 5435, Email: enquiries@stat.org.uk, www.stat.org.uk

Feldenkrais

Feldenkrais Guild UK, PO Box 370, London N10 3XA; Tel: (07000) 785506, Email: enquiries@feldenkrais.co.uk, www.feldenkrais.co.uk

Feldenkrais International Training Centre Ltd, PO Box 1207, Hove, East Sussex BN3 2GG; Tel: (01273) 327406, Fax: (01273) 725299, Email: garetnewell@compuserve.com, www.feldenkrais.co.uk

Massage

British Federation of Massage Practitioners, 78 Meadow Street, Preston, Lancashire PR1 1TS; Tel: (01772) 881063, Fax: (01772) 881063, Email: Jolanta@Jolanta.co.uk, www.jolanta.co.uk

British Massage Therapy Council, 17 Rymers Lane, Oxford OX4 3JU; Tel: (01865) 774123, Fax: (01865) 774123, Email: Infor@bmtc.co.uk, www.bmtc.co.uk

Pilates

Pilates Foundation, 80 Camden Road, London E17 7NF; Tel: (07071) 781859, Fax: (0520) 7586 4579, www.pilatesfoundation.com

Backlund Pilates, 121 Dawes Road, London SW6 7DU; Tel: (020) 7386 7040, Email: info@backlundpilates.com, www.backlundpilates.com

Belsize Studio, 5 McCrone Mews, Belsize Lane, London NW3 5BG; Tel: (020) 7431 6223, Fax: (020) 7813 3372, Email: pilates@belsizestudio.com, www.belsizestudio.com

Brigid McCarthy Pilates Studio, 16 Canning Street, Edinburgh EH3 8EG; Tel: (0131) 221 1131, Email: pilates@breathemail.net, www.mccarthypilates.co.uk

Pilates Off the Square, 4 Mandeville Place, London W1U 2BG; Tel: (020) 7935 8505, Email: pilatesclinic@hotmail.com, www.PilatesOffTheSquare.co.uk

Pilates & Yoga Movement Studio, Quex Road Methodist Church, Kingsgate Road, Kilburn, London NW6 4PR; Tel: (020) 7624 3948, Email: enquiries@pilatesyoga.com, www.pilatesyoga.com

Southeast Pilates Exercise Centre, 969–973 London Road, Leigh-on-Sea, SS9 3LB; Tel: (011702) 710 273, Email: gapb@totalreform.freeserve.co.uk

T'ai Chi

British Council for Chinese Martial Arts, c/o 110 Frensham Drive, Stodkingford, Nuneaton, Warwickshire CV10 9QL; Tel: (02476) 394642, www.bccma.org.uk

Herts Long Fei Taijiquan Association, 16 Blakes Way, Welwyn, Hertfordshire AL6 9RE; Tel: (01438) 718769, www.longfei-taiji.co.uk

Practical Tai Chi Chuan, 9 Ashfield Road, London N14 7LA; Tel: (020) 8368 6815, www.taichichuan.co.uk

T'ai Chi UK, 25 Arrol House, Rockinham Street, London SE1 6QJ; Tel: (020) 7407 4775, Email: info@taichiuk.co.uk, www.taichiuk.co.uk

The Tai Chi Union, 1 Littlemill Drive, Balmoral Gardens, Crookston, Glasgow G53 7GE; Tel: (0141) 810 3482, Fax: (0141) 810 3741, www.taichiunion.com

Yoga

British School of Yoga, Stanhope Square, Holsworthy, Devon EX22 6PF ; Tel: (01409) 271432, Fax: (0207) 287 3348, Email: info@bsygroup.co.uk, www.bsygroup.co.uk

British Wheel of Yoga, 1 Hamilton Place, Boston Road, Sleaford, Lincolnshire NG34 7ES; Tel: (01529) 306851

Iyengar Yoga Institute, 223a Randolph Avenue, London W9 1NL; Tel: (020) 7624 3080, Fax: (020) 73372 2726, Email: office@iyi.org.uk, www.iyi.org.uk

Hairdressing

British Association of Beauty Therapy and Cosmetology, BABTAC House, 70 Eastgate Street, Gloucester GL1 1QN; Tel: (01452) 421114, Fax: (01452) 421110

Caribbean and Afro Society of Hairdressers (CASH), 42 North Cross Road, London SE22; Tel: (020) 8299 2859

Confederation of International Beauty Therapy and Cosmetology (CIBTEC), BABTAC House, 70 Eastgate Street, Gloucester GL1 1QN; Tel: (01452) 421114, Fax: (01452) 421110

Film and Television Freelance Training, 4th Floor, Warwick House, 9 Warwick Street, London W1R 5RA; Tel: (020) 7734 5141, www.ft2.org.uk

Guild of Hairdressers, Unit 1E, Redbrook Business Park, Wilthorpe Road, Barnsley S75 1JN; Tel: (01226) 786555, www.hairguild.org

Hairdressing and Beauty Industry Authority (HABIA), Fraser House, Nether Hall Road, Doncaster DN1 2PH; Tel: (01302) 380000, Fax: (01302) 380028, Email: enquiries@habia.org.uk, www.habia.org.uk

Hairdressing Council, 12 David House, 45 High Street, South Norwood, London SE25 6AJ; Tel: (020) 8771 6205, Fax: (020) 8653 9627, Email: registrar@haircouncil.org.uk, www.haircouncil.demon.uk

Hairdressing Employers Association, 10 Coldbath Square, London EC1R 5HL; Tel: (020) 7833 0633; Tel: (020) 7833 2192, beh@heabaphe.idps.co.uk

Hairdressing Trainers Organization, 28 Roseberry Avenue, Benfleet, Essex SS7 4HJ; Tel: (01268) 759990, www.essexsalons.co.uk

Hairdressing Training Board (Scotland), PO Box 14425, Cupar, KY15 4YE; Tel: (01334) 650102, Fax: (01334) 650102, Email: regionl@legend.co.uk

National Hairdressers Federation, 11 Goldington Road, Bedford MK40 3JY, (01234) 360332, Email: nhf@tgis.co.uk, www.nhfuk.com

Skillset National Training Organization, 2nd Floor, 103 Dean Street, London W1V 5RA; Tel: (020) 7534 5300, Fax: (020) 7534 5333, Email: info@skillset.org, www.skillset.org

Steiner Training Ltd, 92 Uxbridge Road, Harrow Weald, Middlesex HA3 6BZ; Tel: (020) 8909 5016

Vocational Training Charitable Trust, Unit 11, Brickfield Trading Estate, Chandlers Ford, Hampshire SO53 4DR; Tel: (023) 8027 1733, Fax: (023) 8027 0566

Trichology

The Institute of Trichologists, 5 Belsford Court, Nottingham NG16 1JW; Tel: (08706) 070602, Fax: (0115) 938 4303, Email: trichologists@ambernet.co.uk, www.ambernet.co.uk

12 Further reading

Aromatherapy

Price, S (1987) *Practical Aromatherapy: How to Use Essential Oils to Restore Vitality*, Thorsons second edn

Whichello Brown, D (1996) *Teach Yourself Aromatherapy*, Hodder Headline

Beauty

Working in Beauty and Hairdressing booklet, Careers and Occupational Information Centre (COIC)

Career Routes: The official guide to careers in hairdressing and beauty therapy, HABIA

The Guild of Professional Beauty Therapists publishes a training directory and a magazine entitled *Guild News*, which sets out the latest techniques in beauty therapy.

Fitness

Working in Sport and Fitness (1996) Careers and Occupational Information Centre (COIC) (Department for Education and Employment)

FitPro Magazine – for studio co-ordinators and group fitness instructors, FitPro

Fitness Network Magazine – for personal trainers, gym instructors, health club and leisure centre staff and management, FitPro

Fyfe, L (1998) *Careers in Sport*, Kogan Page

Training and Educational Courses in Sport and Recreation (Annual publication), Sports Council

Sport and Recreation: How to Get In – A Guide for Students, SPRITO

Fitness therapies

Brown, L (1999) *Teach Yourself Alternative Medicine*, Hodder Headline

Craze, R (1996) *Teach Yourself Alexander Technique*, Hodder Headline

Feldenkrais, M (1972) *Awareness Through Movement: Health Exercises for Personal Growth*, Harper & Row

Fulder, S (1996) *The Handbook of Alternative and Complementary Medicine*, Vermilion, third edn

Iyengar, B K S (2001) *Light on Yoga*, Thorsons, new edn

Leibowitz, J and Connington, B (1991) *The Alexander Technique*, Souvenir Press

Robinson, L and Thomson, G (1998) *Body Control The Pilates Way*, Pan Books

Woodham, A and Peters Dr D, (1997) *Encyclopaedia of Complementary Medicine*, Dorling Kindersley

Hairdressing

Working in Beauty and Hairdressing booklet, Careers and Occupational Information Centre (COIC)

Career Routes: The official guide to careers in hairdressing and beauty therapy, HABIA

Index